# Inflammatory Bowel Diseases

## A Clinician's Guide

*Ashwin N. Ananthakrishnan MD MPH*

*Assistant Professor of Medicine*
*Harvard Medical School*
*Director*
*Crohn's and Colitis Center*
*Massachusetts General Hospital*
*Boston, MA, USA*

*Ramnik J. Xavier MD*

*Kurt Isselbacher Professor of Medicine*
*Harvard Medical School;*
*Chief of Gastroenterology*
*Massachusetts General Hospital;*
*Institute Member*
*Broad Institute of MIT and Harvard*
*Boston, MA, USA*

*Daniel K. Podolsky MD*

*President*
*University of Texas Southwestern Medical Center*
*Professor of Internal Medicine*
*University of Texas Southwestern Medical School*
*Dallas, TX, USA*

**WILEY** Blackwell

This edition first published 2017 © 2017 by John Wiley & Sons Ltd

*Registered Office*
John Wiley & Sons Ltd, The Atrium, Southern Gate, Chichester, West Sussex, PO19 8SQ, UK

*Editorial Offices*
9600 Garsington Road, Oxford, OX4 2DQ, UK
The Atrium, Southern Gate, Chichester, West Sussex, PO19 8SQ, UK.
111 River Street, Hoboken, NJ 07030-5774, USA

For details of our global editorial offices, for customer services and for information about how to apply for permission to reuse the copyright material in this book please see our website at www.wiley.com/wiley-blackwell

*Library of Congress Cataloging-in-Publication Data*
Names: Ananthakrishnan, Ashwin N., author. | Xavier, Ramnik J., author. | Podolsky, Daniel Kalman, author.
Title: Inflammatory bowel diseases : a clinician's guide / Ashwin N. Ananthakrishnan, Ramnik J. Xavier,
    Daniel K. Podolsky.
Description: Chichester, West Sussex, UK ; Hoboken, NJ : John Wiley & Sons, Inc., 2017. |
    Includes bibliographical references and index.
Identifiers: LCCN 2017001705 (print) | LCCN 2017002995 (ebook) | ISBN 9781119077602 (cloth) |
    ISBN 9781119077619 (pdf) | ISBN 9781119077626 (epub)
Subjects: | MESH: Inflammatory Bowel Diseases
Classification: LCC RC862.I53 (print) | LCC RC862.I53 (ebook) | NLM WI 420 | DDC 616.3/44–dc23
LC record available at https://lccn.loc.gov/2017001705

A catalogue record for this book is available from the British Library.

Wiley also publishes its books in a variety of electronic formats. Some content that appears in print may not be available in electronic books.

Cover images: The image fifth from the left (inset) is reproduced with permission of Vikram Deshpande MD. (See the caption for figure 2.4 for more details.) All other images are courtesy of the authors.

Set in 10/12pt Warnock by SPi Global, Pondicherry, India
Printed and bound in Singapore by Markono Print Media Pte Ltd

1   2017

# Contents

# Preface

Inflammatory bowel diseases (IBDs), comprising Crohn's disease (CD) and ulcerative colitis (UC), are complex diseases that often have their onset during young adulthood. They have a protracted course characterized by periods of remission and relapse, and frequently result in hospitalization, surgery, and continued morbidity. Importantly, they also exert a significant impact on the individuals' health-related quality of life and work productivity. Physicians caring for patients with IBD encounter varied and often complex challenges. The importance of optimal decision-making for the welfare of the patient cannot be overstated.

This book was developed to serve as a resource for practicing physicians, allied healthcare providers, and trainees who care for patients with Crohn's disease and ulcerative colitis. Although exhaustive textbooks are available, this new handbook aims to provide a concise understanding of these disorders and practical guidance on approaches to diagnosis and treatment. Care of patients with IBD is integral to the practice of gastroenterology and frequently also encountered by internists, surgeons, pediatricians, and other physicians, in addition to nurses and other caregivers.

The past two decades have witnessed a significant revolution both in our understanding of the pathogenesis behind these complex diseases and in the availability of therapeutic options that have enhanced the ability to achieve clinical and endoscopic remission. Facilitated by advances in sequencing tools and analytic methods, we now recognize that these diseases arise as a result of a dysregulated immune response to intestinal microflora in a genetically susceptible individual. Over 150 genes have been identified that contribute to the pathogenesis of these disease, influencing innate and adaptive immune responses and integrity of the intestinal barrier. The intestinal microflora demonstrate a dysbiotic pattern with reduced diversity and altered abundance of pro- and anti-inflammatory bacterial species. Therapeutic paradigms have evolved with our understanding of the benefit of effective treatment early in the course of disease and the role of combination therapy to reduce immunogenicity and increase the likelihood of sustained response. Whereas therapy for IBD was initially restricted to broad, non-selective immunosuppressive therapy, emerging treatments increasingly target specific inflammatory pathways such as tumor necrosis factor α, adhesion molecules, and the IL-23 pathway. Yet this scientific and therapeutic revolution has made the management of these diseases more complex than ever before.

*Part I* describes the epidemiology and pathogenesis of IBD, including the role of genetics, the environment, and the gut microbiome. We discuss the clinical features and procedures that aid in establishing a diagnosis of Crohn's disease and ulcerative colitis. We also discuss the various manifestations of

IBD that occur outside the intestine and are a source of morbidity to a significant fraction of patients. We discuss the evolution of these diseases towards more complicated behavior and identify relevant risk factors.

*Part II* discusses each of the classes of therapeutic agents used for the management of IBD, and systematically examines the efficacy of each class in the treatment of patients with ulcerative colitis or Crohn's disease. We also discuss the safety of each category and review newer therapeutic modalities such as those aimed at the microbiome.

*Part III* presents practical algorithms for the medical and surgical management of ulcerative colitis and Crohn's disease, stratifying by severity and extent of involvement. We also review the disease-specific complications for each IBD subtype and the management of these complications.

*Part IV* reviews some special clinical considerations in the management of these diseases, including the role of nutrition and dietary therapies, and two commonly encountered clinical scenarios – the management of IBD during pregnancy and in children – ending with a discussion of transition of care.

Throughout this book, learning is facilitated by practical take-home points in each chapter and patient-centered questions reviewing the material covered in each chapter. Overall, we hope that this guide will enable clinicians to provide the best help to their patients with IBD through the many challenges that they may face.

Section I

**Pathogenesis and Clinical Features**

# 1

# Epidemiology and Pathogenesis

## Clinical Take Home Messages

- Inflammatory bowel diseases (IBDs) have a peak incidence in the second through fourth decades of life but may have their onset at any age.
- Most studies have suggested comparable rates of incidence across both genders but risk of disease varies among ethnic populations, e.g., higher frequency in the Ashkenazi Jewish population.
- Family history is the strongest risk factor for development of IBD. At least 163 distinct genetic polymorphisms have been described in association with Crohn's disease (CD) or ulcerative colitis (UC) but explain less than one-quarter of the variance in risk for either disease.
- Disease risk alleles highlight the importance of various genetic pathways in the pathogenesis of these diseases, including innate immunity, adaptive immune response, intestinal barrier function, and pathogen sensing and response. However, polymorphisms at these loci have not been consistently associated with natural history and phenotype of IBD except for correlation between NOD2 polymorphisms and ileal fibrostenosing CD.
- Several environmental factors may influence risk of disease and subsequent natural history. The most robust data support an effect of cigarette smoking (increasing risk of CD and reducing risk of UC), but other factors including diet, stress and depression, antibiotic exposure, environmental hygiene, vitamin D, physical activity, and hormones may play a role.

## Epidemiology

Crohn's disease (CD) and ulcerative colitis (UC) are chronic, immunologically mediated diseases. They may occur at any age but most often have an onset during young adulthood and a protracted course characterized by remissions and relapses over the course of their natural history. They affect an estimated 2.2 million individuals in Europe and 1.5 million in the United States.

The incidence and prevalence appear to be increasing in areas of the world where historically rates have been far lower than found in Northern Europe and North America, such as Asia. The peak age of onset of CD is between 20 and 30 years whereas UC has a peak incidence a decade later between the ages of 30 and 40 years. However, up to 15% of patients may have their first presentation of inflammatory bowel disease (IBD) after the age of 65 years,

*Inflammatory Bowel Diseases: A Clinician's Guide*, First Edition. Ashwin N. Ananthakrishnan, Ramnik J. Xavier, and Daniel K. Podolsky.
© 2017 John Wiley & Sons Ltd. Published 2017 by John Wiley & Sons Ltd.

and a bimodal pattern of incidence with a second smaller peak in the sixth and seventh decades of life has been described, particularly for UC. In addition, a subset of patients can manifest IBD at a very early age, less than 2 years old, termed very early-onset IBD (VEOIBD), which is characterized by distinct genetic predisposition and clinical phenotype characterized by treatment refractoriness, severe perianal disease, and response to bone marrow transplant.

The incidence of UC in several countries in the Western Hemisphere is informed by large population-based cohorts tracking secular trends. However, incidence data are lacking from other parts of the world where the emergence of these diseases has been more recent. In North America, the incidence of UC ranges from 0 to 19.2 per 100 000 persons and a similar distribution exists in Europe. CD has a similar incidence, ranging between 0.3 and 12.7 per 100 000 persons in Europe and between 0 and 20.2 per 100 000 persons in North America. Serial estimates of incidence from population-based cohorts dating back to the mid-twentieth century reveal interesting secular trends. In Olmsted County, Minnesota, the incidence of UC rose from 0.6 per 100,000 in 1940–1943 to 8.3 per 100 000 in 1990–1993, with the steepest increase in incidence in the 1970s. CD similarly rose from 1.0 per 100,000 person-years in 1940–1943 to 6.9 cases per 100 000 person-years in 1984–1993. A systematic review of all studies examining trends in disease incidence suggested that over 75% of the studies involving CD and 60% of the studies involving UC identified secular increases in disease incidence. Virtually no study has reported a consistent decrease in incidence in any population over time. Both CD (incidence 0–5.0 per 100 000) and UC (incidence 0.1–6.3 per 100 000) remain relatively uncommon in Asia compared with Western populations. However, increasing incidence, potentially paralleling westernization of life

style, has been found in several Asian countries over the past few decades, including Japan, China, Taiwan, and Korea (Figure 1.1). Interestingly, the incidence for UC generally occurs first, followed a decade later by an increase in the incidence of CD.

There are well-recognized ethnic differences in risk for CD and UC, and less consistently a difference by gender. In most studies, CD and UC occur equally frequently among men and women, although in some studies there is a slight predominance of men among patients with UC (60%) and a predominance of women among those with CD. The incidence of both diseases is more common in the Jewish population; the risk of CD is 3–8-fold that of non-Jews, with a more modest but still elevated risk of UC [1]. The incidence is lower among Sephardic than Ashkenazi Jews and in Israeli than American and European Jews. An international cohort of eight countries in the Asia–Pacific region identified higher incidences of both diseases in Australia than in Asia, but also geographic and ethnic variations within the different countries in Asia [2]. IBD is also uncommon in certain subpopulations even within a high-incidence geographic region such as the First Nations population in Canada and the Aboriginal population in Australia. Within North America, the prevalence of CD and UC was initially reported to be lower in African American and Hispanic populations, but recent data suggest a rising incidence within these populations and an incidence comparable to the lower end of that reported for Caucasians [3]. The risk of IBD varies with migration from a low- to a high-incidence area. Studies in the United Kingdom and Sweden have demonstrated that the risk, particularly of UC, in immigrants from low-incidence countries rapidly approaches the rate in the local population within one or two generations. However, this change in

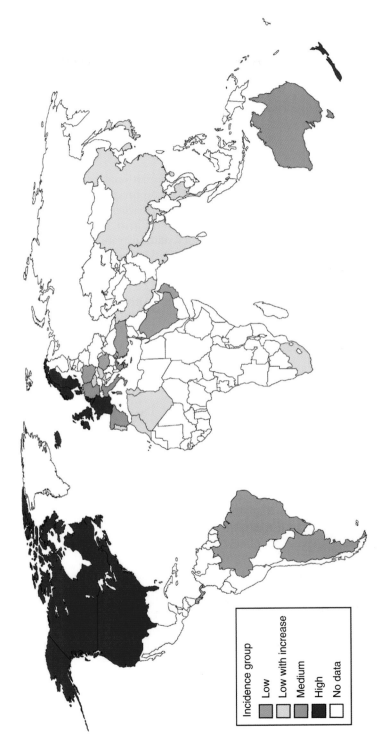

Figure 1.1 Geographic variation in incidence of Crohn's disease and ulcerative colitis. *Source:* Adapted from Cosnes *et al.* 2011 [26]. Reproduced with permission of Elsevier.

risk is dependent on the country of origin. Individuals of South Asian or West Asian origin experience a greater increase in disease risk whereas the risk in those from East Asia remains lower than in the country of residence [4].

## Pathogenesis

The key mechanism underlying the development of IBD appears to be a dysregulated immune response to commensal flora in a genetically susceptible individual (Figure 1.2). Family history is one of the strongest risk factors for the development of disease. Only 10–20% of patients will have an affected first-degree relative. However, the risk of the offspring developing IBD increases 2–13-fold if one parent is affected. This absolute risk can be as high as 36% if both parents are affected. The concordance of disease is greater in

monozygotic twins (30–35%) than dizygotic twins, also supporting an important role for genetics in these diseases. However, genetic mutations alone are not sufficient for disease except in the rare VEOIBD owing to high-penetrance mutations involving the interleukin (IL)-10 receptor.

### Genetics

An international consortium has identified 163 common risk loci for IBD. Most loci are shared between both diseases; 30 loci are distinctly associated with CD whereas 23 loci demonstrate genome-wide significant association with UC alone. These loci together explain only 13.6% of the variance in risk of CD and 7.5% of the variance in risk for UC. Although most common loci demonstrate an effect in the same direction, two loci demonstrate divergent effects. *NOD2* and *PTPN22* polymorphisms are associated

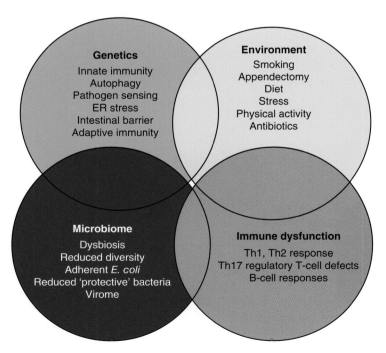

**Figure 1.2** Inflammatory bowel disease develops as a result of a complex interplay between genetics, the microbiome, immunologic dysregulation, and the external environment.

with an increased risk of CD but are inversely associated with UC. Several of the loci are also implicated in other autoimmune diseases, including psoriasis and celiac disease, suggesting considerable sharing of pathogenic pathways across various autoimmune or inflammatory diseases. Although the spectrum of immunologic disruption as a consequence of these genetic polymorphisms is wide, several pathways emerge as being important in the development of IBD. These include the innate immunity, autophagy, adaptive immune responses, pathogen sensing, maintenance of the intestinal barrier through the mucous layer and epithelial integrity, and response to oxidative stress. Several genes may influence the same pathway. For example, *HNF4A*, *MUC19*, *CDH1*, and *GNA12* all influence intestinal barrier integrity whereas *NOD2*, *ATG16L1*, *IRGM*, and *LRRK2* affect autophagy. The pathways may act in isolation, in combination with each other, or in conjunction with environmental insults. For example, the functional consequences of autophagy defects on Paneth cell function are triggered by infection with the Norovirus. The identified genetic polymorphisms also highlight the substantial evolutionary conversation between pathways that are important in the development of autoimmune diseases, but also play an important role in mediating responses to infections. For example, polymorphisms in the vitamin D receptor (*VDR*) or *SLC11A1*, both linked to IBD, are also associated with increased risk of *Mycobacterium tuberculosis* infection, and *NOD2* and *LRRK2* polymorphisms are associated with leprosy. Some of the IBD risk variants (*STAT3*, *CARD9*) are also associated with primary immunodeficiency states and may predispose to recurrent bacterial or fungal infections.

*NOD2* was the first genetic variant to be associated with CD [5, 6]. It functions as an intracellular sensor of the peptidoglycan muramyl dipeptide (MDP), a component of bacterial cell walls. Stimulation of *NOD2* by MDP results in activation of a cascade of inflammatory pathways involving nuclear factor-κB (NF-κB) and mitogen-activated protein (MAP) kinase signaling resulting in the production of inflammatory cytokines including tumor necrosis factor alpha (TNF-α) and IL-1β. Three common polymorphisms – Arg702Trp, Gly908Arg, and Leu1007fsX1008 – and five rare variants in *NOD2* have been identified through deep sequencing. *NOD2* also activates T-cell responses through MDP-independent mechanisms. Despite *NOD2* variants being associated with the greatest relative risk of CD, their presence alone is not sufficient for disease as up to 30% of individuals of European ancestry may carry such variants. In addition, *NOD2* has not been consistently associated with CD in non-European populations.

Variants in genes whose products contribute to autophagy, a cellular process involved in intracellular microbial clearance and degradation of cytosolic contents, have also been associated with CD, most notably variants of *ATG16L1* and *IRGM*. In addition to their independent effect, autophagy variants may influence susceptibility to environmental triggers through a "two-hit" hypothesis. This was highlighted in an elegant study in which the defects in Paneth cell structure and function in ATG16L1 knockout mice were exaggerated in the setting of murine Norovirus infection [7].

Adaptive immune responses, through both T- and B-lymphocytes, play an important role in the pathogenesis of IBD. In the setting of active inflammation, naive T cells are activated and differentiate into Th1, Th2, or Th17 cells depending on the influence of different cytokines [8, 9]. Th1 cells, initially thought to be key in the pathogenesis of Crohn's disease, produce TNF-α and interferon gamma (IFN-γ) along with other cytokines that activate macrophages, lead to epithelial cell apoptosis, and induce differentiation of stromal myofibroblasts, which, through the production of matrix metalloproteinases, result in degradation of the extracellular matrix. In contrast, Th2 cells produce IL-13, which increases intestinal permeability and induces epithelial apoptosis [8, 9].

A relatively recently described class of helper T cells – Th17 cells – produce IL-17A, IL-21, and IL-22, which aid in neutrophil recruitment and inflammation through activation of NF-κB and MAPK pathways [8, 9]. Several other cell types also appear to play important roles in the pathogenesis of IBD. The innate lymphoid cell (ILC) is a newly described effector cell subtype that makes IFN-γ (group 1 ILC), IL-5 and IL-13 (group 2 ILCs), or IL-17, IL-22, and IFN-γ (group 3 ILCs). Group 3 ILCs in particular appear to play an important role in inducing colitis through an IL-23R/IL-22-dependent mechanism. In an animal model, $RAG^{-/-}$ mice developed colitis after injection of CD40 ligand (CD40L), but only in the presence of innate lymphoid cells [10].

Trafficking of leukocytes to the small intestine and colon, mediated through chemoattractants, chemokine receptors, and adhesion molecules, plays an important role in homing of lymphocytes into gut-associated lymphoid tissues at the site of inflammation [11]. For example, the mucosal vascular addressin cell adhesion molecule 1 (MADCAM1), expressed on the high endothelial venules of Peyer's patches and on the venules of small intestine and colon, is a receptor for the α4β7 integrin and facilitates migration of leukocytes to Peyer's patches and sites of intestinal inflammation [11].

The rapid pace of discovery in the field of genetics and immunopathogenesis of these diseases has contributed to the development of existing and emerging therapeutics and highlighted novel effective modalities of action. Monoclonal antibodies to TNF-α, reviewed in detail in subsequent chapters, are among the most effective existing treatments for both CD and UC. Recognition of the importance of the IL-17/IL-23 pathway in IBD led to the development of an antibody targeting the p40 subunit of IL-12/IL-23, ustekinumab, that is already in use for the treatment of psoriasis and shows promise in the management of CD. Leukocyte migration has been targeted by several drug categories, including monoclonal antibodies such as natalizumab and vedolizumab, and also small-molecule inhibitors. The direct implication of genotype in guiding a personalized approach to diagnosis or therapy is less well established. NOD2 mutations are associated with ileal location or fibrostenosing CD. None of the other genetic mutations have been consistently predictive of natural history or response to therapy, although panels comprising multiple genes show a modest ability to predict therapy response.

### Microbiome

Several lines of evidence support an important role for the intestinal microbiome in the pathogenesis of IBD. Mice genetically predisposed to develop colitis, such as $IL10^{-/-}$ or $TCR\alpha^{-/-}$, either do not develop colitis in germ-free conditions, or develop only attenuated inflammation (*SAMP1/yit* or $IL2^{-/-}$ mice). Defects in pattern recognition receptors such as Toll-like receptors result in attenuation of the colitis. Several polymorphisms important in the development of IBD, for example *NOD2* and *ATG16L1*, are key for the recognition of patterns from luminal microbial antigens and activation of innate immune responses in response to such stimulation. Polymorphisms at these loci result in aberrant Paneth cell function and impaired production of antimicrobial peptides, further highlighting the importance of luminal microbial antigenic stimulation. Clinically, in patients with CD, exposure to the fecal stream is essential for the development of postoperative recurrence after intestinal resection [12, 13].

The normal adult human microbiome contains $10^{13}-10^{14}$ bacterial cells and an estimated 1000 different bacterial species. The largest microbial community in the human intestine is Bacteroidetes with a smaller proportion of Firmicutes. Other important groups occurring at a lower frequency are Proteobacteria, Actinobacteria, Fusobacteria, and Verrucomicrobia. There is substantial inter-individual variation in the intestinal microbiome, which attains stability after the first 2–4 years of life. The intestinal microbiota is also susceptible to the effect of external environmental influences, most prominently diet and antibiotic exposure.

Three dominant patterns of gut microbial changes are apparent in patients with IBD. First, there is an overall reduction in diversity and abundance of gut microbiota in patients with IBD compared with controls. Mucosal biopsies in IBD demonstrate a reduced abundance of Firmicutes and Bacteroidetes and an increase in Proteobacteria and Actinobacteria [14, 15]. Second, specific subphenotypes of IBD may demonstrate an increase in some pathogenic microbes. Specifically, enteroadherent *Escherichia coli* is found at a greater frequency in ileal lesions of patients with CD than with UC or in healthy controls [16]. Third, patients with IBD may demonstrate a reduced frequency of bacteria, which may be important in conferring protection from intestinal inflammation. For example, individuals with IBD have reduced levels of short-chain fatty acids in stool, pointing to the potential role of Ruminococcaceae, which are important butyrate producers. They also have reduced abundance of *Faecalibacterium prausnitzii*, a bacterium belonging to the Clostridiales family. Furthermore, the prevalence of *F. prausnitzii* correlates inversely with likelihood of endoscopic recurrence of CD following intestinal resection and supernatants from *F. prausnitzii* cultures ameliorate colitis in animal models [17, 18]. In addition to the above variations in composition of the gut microbiome, there are also differences in functional pathways between IBD and healthy individuals, including those mediating response to oxidative stress, and a decrease in carbohydrate and amino acid biosynthesis [19]. However, bacteria may not be the sole components of the gut microbiome influencing susceptibility to IBD. Viral infections, particularly in the context of specific genetic polymorphisms, may act as triggers for intestinal inflammation and disruption of immune function [7]. Fungal diversity may be increased in patients with IBD.

### Environmental Triggers

Several environmental factors appear to influence the risk of and natural history of IBD. Harries *et al.* [20] first noted that patients with UC were less frequently smokers than healthy individuals. Several studies since have replicated this association and demonstrated an increased risk of CD among current and former smokers. In contrast to the inverse association between current smoking and UC, smoking cessation is associated with a twofold increase in risk of UC that is apparent within 2–5 years of cessation and may persist for up to 20 years. Passive smoking has a similar direction of effect. The effect of smoking is not uniform in all populations and may be dependent on ethnicity and gender. Women are more susceptible to the adverse effects of smoking on IBD whereas men have a greater magnitude of the protective effect of cigarette smoke on UC. Smoking exerts an influence on natural history of disease similar to its effect on incident disease. Current smokers have more aggressive CD with a greater need for immunosuppression, a higher likelihood of surgery, and increased risk of recurrence after resection. In contrast, in UC, smoking is associated with a milder course and reduced likelihood of surgery. It is unclear which substance(s) within tobacco smoke are responsible for these effects. Trials with nicotine-based agents do not ameliorate disease in patients with UC. A similar interesting divergent direction of effect is seen for appendectomy. When performed before the age of 20 years and for inflammatory appendicitis, it is associated with a reduced risk of UC [21]. In contrast, it does not confer similar protection against CD and may be associated with an increased risk.

Given the central role of the microbiome in disease pathogenesis and the strong influence of long- and short-term diet on gut composition, it is plausible that diet plays a role in the predisposition to developing IBD or influences subsequent natural history. However, high-quality prospective data informing such associations are lacking. The most consistent dietary association described is an inverse relationship between fruits, vegetables, or fiber intake and risk of CD. Several plausible mechanisms support this association. Soluble fiber may prevent bacterial transmigration through the epithelium and modify the composition of gut microbiota. Specific dietary substances may be ligands for the aryl hydrocarbon receptor, which plays a role in ameliorating gut inflammation. Dietary fat may increase the risk of UC although the data are less consistent and many studies have shown no effect. However, in animal models, a high milk fat diet resulted in expansion of pathobionts in the gut and more severe colitis. n-3 polyunsaturated fatty acids such as are found in fish oil have been inversely associated with risk of UC, although therapeutic interventions modifying their intake have yielded mostly unsuccessful results in both CD and UC. Studies have also demonstrated substantial heterogeneity in susceptibility to symptomatic exacerbations in response to the intake of specific foods. Therapeutically, elemental diet is effective in inducing remission in pediatric CD but is poorly tolerated over the long term. Several other elimination diets have been proposed but there is a lack evidence in support of efficacy.

Other environmental influences associated with risk of IBD include antibiotic exposure, low vitamin D, sleep, stress and depression, physical activity, hormone use, non-steroidal anti-inflammatory drugs (NSAIDs) and aspirin, breastfeeding, environmental hygiene, and exposure to animals in childhood. Although offering intriguing insights into disease pathogenesis, few of these have been translated into interventions to benefit individuals with established disease. Normalization of vitamin D levels in patients with deficiency is associated with a reduction in risk of subsequent surgeries, and vitamin D supplementation may reduce the likelihood of relapses. Interventions targeting stress and depression may improve psychological quality of life but have a variable impact on actual clinical disease activity. Enteric infections, in particular *Clostridium difficile* infection, are frequent triggers of relapses in those with established IBD and should be sought for in the setting of unexplained clinical activity (Table 1.1). Although ascertaining exposure to some of these potential triggers at the time of disease exacerbation is reasonable, with the exception of smoking cessation in those with established CD, systematic efforts to modify these risk factors with the aim of influencing overall disease activity cannot be recommended due to lack of high-quality interventional studies.

Table 1.1 Effect of environmental risk factors on risk of development of Crohn's disease or ulcerative colitis.

| Environmental factor | Crohn's disease | Ulcerative colitis |
|---|---|---|
| *Smoking* | | |
|     Current smoking | Increased risk | Decreased risk |
|     Former smoking | Increased risk | Increased risk |
|     Appendectomy | Equivocal | Decreased risk |
| *Diet* | | |
|     Dietary fiber, Fruits, vegetables | Reduces risk | No effect |
|     Dietary fat | Equivocal | High n-3 polyunsaturated fats may reduce risk whereas n-6 fats may be associated with increased risk<br>Saturated fat diet (particularly milk fat) may be associated with increased risk |
|     Protein | Equivocal | Equivocal. May increase risk |
|     Zinc | Decreased risk | No effect |
| Stress, depression | Increased risk | Increased risk |
| NSAIDs, aspirin | Increased risk | Increased risk |
| Low vitamin D levels | Increased risk | No effect |
| Antibiotic use | Increased risk | Increased risk |
| History of being breastfed | Decreased risk | Decreased risk |

## Case Studies and Multiple Choice Questions

1  John is a 26-year-old male who presented to his gastroenterologist with complaints of diarrhea and rectal bleeding of 4 months' duration. He has no extraintestinal symptoms. He has no family history of IBD. A colonoscopy is performed and reveals erythema, granularity, friability, and erosions consistent with left-sided ulcerative colitis. Which of the following factors if present in John's history is associated with an increased risk of ulcerative colitis?

  A  Increased intake of dietary fiber.
  B  A history of appendectomy at age 9 years for appendicitis.
  C  Current smoking of one pack per day.
  D  Smoking cessation 2 years prior to diagnosis.

2  The proportion of patients with IBD who will have at least one affected first-degree relative with Crohn's disease or ulcerative colitis is

  A  0–5%.
  B  10–20%.
  C  50–60%.
  D  80–90%.

3  Which of the following changes in the gut microbiome have *not* been described in patients with IBD?

  A  Increased frequency of enteroinvasive *Escherichia coli*.
  B  Reduced diversity of gut microbiota.
  C  Reduced abundance of bacteria belonging to the phylum Firmicutes.
  D  Greater abundance of *Faecalibacterium prausnitzii*.

4  The known 163 common single-nucleotide polymorphisms that modify risk of Crohn's disease or ulcerative colitis explain what proportion of the variance in risk for each disease?

  A  8% of the variance in UC and 14% of the variance in CD.
  B  22% of the variance in UC and 48% of the variance in CD.
  C  60% of the variance in UC and 30% of the variance in CD.
  D  5% of the variance in UC and 20% of the variance in CD.

# References

1 Fireman, Z., Grossman, A., Lilos, P., *et al.* (1989) Epidemiology of Crohn's disease in the Jewish population of central Israel, 1970–1980. *American Journal of Gastroenterology*, **84**(3), 255–258.

2 Ng, S.C., Tang, W., Ching, J.Y., *et al.* (2013) Incidence and phenotype of inflammatory bowel disease based on results from the Asia–Pacific Crohn's and Colitis Epidemiology Study. *Gastroenterology*, **145**(1), 158–165.e2.

3 Hou, J.K., El-Serag, H., and Thirumurthi, S. (2009) Distribution and manifestations of inflammatory bowel disease in Asians, Hispanics, and African Americans: a systematic review. *American Journal of Gastroenterology*, **104**(8), 2100–2109.

4 Li, X., Sundquist, J., Hemminki, K., and Sundquist, K. (2011) Risk of inflammatory bowel disease in first- and second-generation immigrants in Sweden: a nationwide follow-up study. *Inflammatory Bowel Diseases*, **17**(8), 1784–1791.

5 Hugot, J.P., Chamaillard, M., Zouali, H., *et al.* (2001) Association of NOD2 leucine-rich repeat variants with susceptibility to Crohn's disease. *Nature*, **411**(6837), 599–603.

6 Ogura, Y., Bonen, D.K., Inohara, N., *et al.* (2001) A frameshift mutation in NOD2 associated with susceptibility to Crohn's disease. *Nature*, **411**(6837), 603–606.

7 Cadwell, K., Patel, K.K., Maloney, N.S., *et al.* (2010) Virus-plus-susceptibility gene interaction determines Crohn's disease gene Atg16L1 phenotypes in intestine. *Cell*, **141**(7), 1135–1145.

8 Wallace, K.L., Zheng, L.B., Kanazawa, Y., and Shih, D.Q. (2014) Immunopathology of inflammatory bowel disease. *World Journal of Gastroenterology*, **20**(1), 6–21.

9 Geremia, A., Biancheri, P., Allan, P., *et al.* (2014) Innate and adaptive immunity in inflammatory bowel disease. *Autoimmunity Reviews*, **13**(1), 3–10.

10 Buonocore, S., Ahern, P.P., Uhlig, H.H., *et al.* (2010) Innate lymphoid cells drive interleukin-23-dependent innate intestinal pathology. *Nature*, **464**(7293), 1371–1375.

11 Habtezion, A., Nguyen, L.P., Hadeiba, H., and Butcher, E.C. (2016) Leukocyte trafficking to the small intestine and colon. *Gastroenterology*, **150**(2), 340–354.

12 Rutgeerts, P., Goboes, K., Peeters, M., *et al.* (1991) Effect of faecal stream diversion on recurrence of Crohn's disease in the neoterminal ileum. *Lancet*, **338**(8770), 771–774.

13 D'Haens, G.R., Geboes, K., Peeters, M., *et al.* (1998) Early lesions of recurrent Crohn's disease caused by infusion of intestinal contents in excluded ileum. *Gastroenterology*, **114**(2), 262–267.

14 Frank, D.N., St. Amand, A.L., Feldman, R.A., *et al.* (2007) Molecular-phylogenetic characterization of microbial community imbalances in human inflammatory bowel diseases. *Proceedings of the National Academy of Sciences of the United States of America*, **104**(34), 13780–13785.

15 Ott, S.J., Musfeldt, M., Wenderoth, D.F., *et al.* (2004) Reduction in diversity of the colonic mucosa associated bacterial microflora in patients with active inflammatory bowel disease. *Gut*, **53**(5), 685–693.

16 Sepehri, S., Khafipour, E., Bernstein, C.N., *et al.* (2011) Characterization of *Escherichia coli* isolated from gut biopsies of newly diagnosed patients with inflammatory bowel disease. *Inflammatory Bowel Diseases*, **17**(7), 1451–1463.

17 Sokol, H., Seksik, P., Furet, J.P., *et al.* (2009) Low counts of *Faecalibacterium prausnitzii* in colitis microbiota. *Inflammatory Bowel Diseases*, **15**(8), 1183–1189.

18 Sokol, H., Pigneur, B., Watterlot, L., *et al.* (2008) *Faecalibacterium prausnitzii* is an anti-inflammatory commensal bacterium identified by gut microbiota analysis of Crohn disease patients. *Proceedings of the National Academy of Sciences of the United States of America*, **105**(43), 16731–16736.

19 Morgan, X.C., Tickle, T.L., Sokol, H., *et al.* (2012) Dysfunction of the intestinal microbiome in inflammatory bowel disease and treatment. *Genome Biology*, **13**(9), R79.

20 Harries, A.D., Baird, A., and Rhodes, J. (1982) Non-smoking: a feature of ulcerative colitis. *British Medical Journal (Clinical Research Edition)*, **284**(6317), 706.

21 Andersson, R.E., Olaison, G., Tysk, C., and Ekbom, A. (2001) Appendectomy and protection against ulcerative colitis. *New England Journal of Medicine*, **344**(11), 808–814.

22 Birrenbach, T. and Bocker, U. (2004) Inflammatory bowel disease and smoking: a review of epidemiology, pathophysiology, and therapeutic implications. *Inflammatory Bowel Diseases*, **10**(6), 848–859.

23 Higuchi, L.M., Khalili, H., Chan, A.T., *et al.* (2012) A prospective study of cigarette smoking and the risk of inflammatory bowel disease in women. *American Journal of Gastroenterology*, **107**(9), 1399–1406.

24 Knights, D., Lassen, K.G., and Xavier, R.J. (2013) Advances in inflammatory bowel disease pathogenesis: linking host genetics and the microbiome. *Gut*, **62**(10), 1505–1510.

25 Jostins, L., Ripke, S., Weersma, R.K., *et al.* (2012) Host–microbe interactions have shaped the genetic architecture of inflammatory bowel disease. *Nature*, **491**(7422), 119–124.

26 Cosnes, J., Gower-Rousseau, C., Seksik, P., and Cortot, A. (2011) Epidemiology and natural history of inflammatory bowel diseases. *Gastroenterology*, **140**(6), 1785–1794.

## Answers to Questions

1   Answer: **D**. Harries *et al*. first noted an inverse association between current smoking and ulcerative colitis [20, 22], a finding that has since been confirmed in several other cohorts. In contrast to the inverse association with current smoking, smoking cessation is associated with an increased risk of UC (compared with never smoked individuals) beginning within 2–5 years after cessation and persisting for up to 20 years after cessation [23].

2   Answer: **B**. Approximately 10–20% of patients with IBD will have at least one affected first-degree relative with IBD.

3   Answer: **D**. The gut microbiome in IBD is characterized by a reduction in diversity, reduced abundance of Firmicutes and Bacteroidetes, and an increase in Proteobacteria and Actinobacteria [24].

A higher abundance of enteroinvasive *E. coli* [termed adherent invasive *E. coli* (AIEC)] has been described in ileal Crohn's disease but not among those with Crohn's colitis or ulcerative colitis. *F. prausnitzii*, a bacterium belonging to the Clostridiales family, is found at a reduced abundance in patients with IBD, correlates inversely with likelihood of endoscopic recurrence in Crohn's disease, and, when administered intragastrically, ameliorates intestinal inflammation in animal models [18].

4   Answer: **A**. Despite advances in genetics having contributed to the identification of at least 163 distinct single-nucleotide polymorphisms that modify the risk of CD or UC, these loci together explain only 13.6% of the variance in risk of CD and 7.5% of the variance in risk for UC [25].

# 2

# Clinical Features and Diagnosis of Crohn's Disease

## Clinical Take Home Messages

- Crohn's disease (CD) may occur anywhere in the gastrointestinal tract and is characterized endoscopically by deep ulcerations and skip lesions, and histologically by transmural inflammation.
- Clinical presentation depends on location and behavior of disease, presence of perianal involvement, and extraintestinal manifestations.
- The hallmark of CD is disease progression from inflammatory to stricturing or penetrating disease behavior. Such evolution is more common in those with small bowel involvement than isolated colonic disease.
- Up to two-thirds of patients with CD require intestinal resection during the course of their disease and half of such patients require a second surgical resection.
- Lower gastrointestinal endoscopy is usually essential to establish a diagnosis but laboratory investigations, serologic markers, and cross-sectional imaging may be supportive to establish disease extent and severity and identify complications.
- Magnetic resonance enterography (MRE) and computed tomography enterography (CTE) have high accuracy in determining active disease and luminal and extraluminal complications, with the former being preferred owing to lack of radiation exposure.

Crohn's disease (CD) is a progressive disease characterized by focal transmural inflammation. It can involve any site in the gastrointestinal tract, from the mouth to the anus. Whereas the inflammation in ulcerative colitis (UC) is diffuse and superficial, the inflammation in CD is often deep and discontinuous, with distinct areas of normal tissue between affected areas, termed "skip lesions" (Table 2.1). In addition, because of the transmural nature of the inflammation, CD often leads to the development of fistulae or strictures. The location and behavior of CD, classified according to the Montreal classification, are important determinants of presenting symptoms and also natural history (Table 2.2). Over three-quarters of patients with CD will have involvement of the distal ileum. Approximately one-third will have ileal involvement alone, half will have both ileal and colonic disease, and one-fifth will have disease restricted to the colon. Half of the patients with colonic CD will have sparing of the

*Inflammatory Bowel Diseases: A Clinician's Guide*, First Edition. Ashwin N. Ananthakrishnan, Ramnik J. Xavier, and Daniel K. Podolsky.
© 2017 John Wiley & Sons Ltd. Published 2017 by John Wiley & Sons Ltd.

**Table 2.1**  Clinical, endoscopic, and histologic findings differentiating Crohn's disease from ulcerative colitis.

| Characteristic | Crohn's disease | Ulcerative colitis |
|---|---|---|
| *Clinical features* | | |
| Gastrointestinal symptoms | Diarrhea, abdominal pain, growth retardation, anemia | Rectal bleeding, diarrhea, tenesmus, urgency |
| Extraintestinal manifestations | Less frequent | More frequent |
| Perianal involvement | Present in one-fifth | Absent |
| Stricturing complications | May be present | Absent |
| Penetrating complications | May be present | Absent |
| Site of involvement | Mouth to anus | Restricted to the colon |
| *Endoscopic findings* | | |
| Distribution of disease | Patchy with skip areas of involvement and intervening normal mucosa | Usually contiguous |
| Rectal involvement | Usually spared | Nearly uniformly involved |
| Ileal involvement | Frequent. Presents as aphthae, ulcerations, strictures | Infrequent. Backwash ileitis presenting as erythema may be seen in a subset |
| Typical features | Deep ulcers, serpiginous ulcers, cobblestoning | Granular, erythematous mucosa with erosions and friability |
| *Histopathologic findings* | | |
| Depth of inflammation | May be transmural | Restricted to mucosa and submucosa |
| Granulomas | Present in up to one-fifth of patients | Usually absent |

**Table 2.2**  The Montreal classification of disease location and behavior in Crohn's disease.

| | | |
|---|---|---|
| Age at diagnosis | A1 | Below 16 years |
| | A2 | Between 17 and 40 years |
| | A3 | Above 40 years |
| Location | L1 | Ileal |
| | L2 | Colonic |
| | L3 | Ileocolonic |
| | L4 | Isolated upper gastrointestinal disease[a] |
| Behavior[b] | B1 | Non-stricturing, non-penetrating |
| | B2 | Stricturing |
| | B3 | Penetrating |

[a] Can be added to L1–L3 if present concomitantly
[b] A perianal disease modifier "p" can be added to B1–B3 when presenting concomitantly.

rectum. One-third of patients will have coexisting perianal disease. It may precede, occur along with, or follow the diagnosis of luminal CD. A smaller proportion of adult patients with CD (5–15%) will have upper gastrointestinal disease, involving the mouth, esophagus, or gastroduodenal region. At the time of diagnosis, most patients will have an inflammatory behavior, with fewer than 10–20% each presenting with stricturing or penetrating complications at diagnosis [1]. However, the majority of patients will develop stricturing or fistulizing complications over the course of time. Extra-intestinal manifestations will be present in conjunction with luminal disease in some patients with CD.

## Clinical Features

The clinical manifestations of CD depend on the disease location and behavior and the coexistence of perianal or extraintestinal disease.

Involvement of the esophagus, stomach, or duodenum with CD, although infrequent, can be severe. Esophageal CD presents as odynophagia or dysphagia, or may mimic gastroesophageal reflux disease. Gastric or duodenal CD may present with dyspepsia, abdominal pain, and post-prandial fullness or as a non-healing ulcer. Gastric outlet obstruction may also occur, resulting in symptoms of early satiety, post-prandial abdominal distension, and vomiting. Rarely, biliary obstruction or duodenobiliary fistula occurs. Refractory ulceration or the presence of ulcerations at an unusual site and in the absence of known risk factors such as the use of non-steroidal anti-inflammatory drugs (NSAIDs) or *Helicobacter pylori* should trigger suspicion for gastroduodenal CD. Jejunoileal CD presents as abdominal pain, diarrhea, or vomiting. Malabsorption may be more common with extensive small bowel involvement.

Particularly in children, weight loss or growth retardation may be a presenting feature. Focal segmental small bowel strictures may present as episodes of partial bowel obstruction. Jejunal disease is also associated with increased likelihood of surgery and obstructive episodes compared with ileal disease [2].

Ileal and ileocecal CD are the most common patterns of involvement and typically present as right lower quadrant abdominal pain and diarrhea, usually without overt bleeding. Sometimes gastrointestinal blood loss may be acute and the presentation may be associated with severe anemia. Patients who develop penetrating complications such as ileocecal abscess may present with more dominant abdominal pain and systemic symptoms such as fever and night sweats. Physical examination may reveal abdominal tenderness and guarding and peritoneal signs. An acute presentation can mimic appendicitis and other infectious causes of diarrhea such as *Yersinia* infection. Sometimes, the symptoms reflect partial small bowel obstruction with crampy abdominal pain occurring after meals, abdominal distension, nausea, and vomiting. Rarely, visible peristalsis may be reported by the patient or seen on physical examination.

Approximately 20% of patients with CD present with isolated colonic involvement that is sometimes difficult to distinguish from UC. Typically, diarrhea is a more dominant feature of CD, with rectal bleeding being less common than in UC. The manifestations of perianal CD can range from fistulae presenting as discharge of mucopus to perianal abscesses presenting as pelvic pain or perianal pain (Figure 2.1). Pelvic sepsis can present as low back pain or with systemic features. Perianal CD may manifest as skin tags or fissures, and the presence of skin tags in someone with colitis should prompt suspicion for CD. Sometimes, perianal disease can be severe and lead to significant scarring and deformity in the perineum.

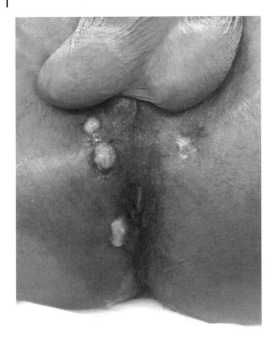

**Figure 2.1** Clinical image of perianal Crohn's disease demonstrating multiple perineal fistulae.

## Disease Course and Natural History

A key feature of CD is progressive bowel damage and a tendency for disease behavior to progress from inflammatory disease to penetrating or stricturing complications. In a cohort of 1199 patients with CD, 60% eventually developed a stricturing or penetrating complication. At 20 years, the rate of inflammatory, stricturing, or penetrating phenotype was 12, 18, and 70%, respectively [1] (Figure 2.2). However, location of disease was an important predictor of evolution. Patients with colonic disease tended to exhibit inflammatory features and remained relatively uncomplicated for many years whereas those with ileal locations progressed to complications faster and in a larger proportion [3]. In a population-based cohort in Olmsted County, Minnesota, at baseline 81% had non-stricturing, non-penetrating disease, 5% had stricturing disease, and 14%

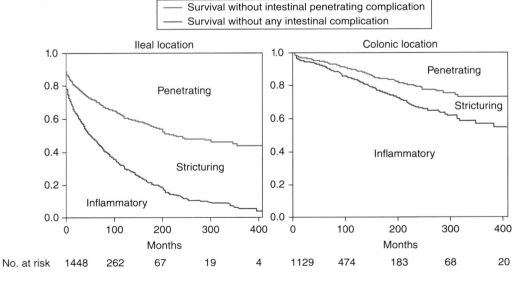

**Figure 2.2** Natural history of Crohn's disease is characterized by progression with an increasing proportion of penetrating and stricturing complications. *Source:* Adapted from Cosnes *et al.* 2011 [3]. Reproduced with permission of Elsevier.

had penetrating disease. However, at 20 years, the cumulative risk of developing stricturing or penetrating complications was 51%, with 66/306 patients changing their behavior within 90 days of diagnosis [4]. In contrast to the evolution in disease behavior, the location of CD tends to be stable over time. Ten years after diagnosis, disease extension to the small bowel in patients with colonic disease, or the colon in patients with small bowel disease at diagnosis, occurs in fewer than 20% of patients [5]. The cumulative risk of perianal fistula 20 years after diagnosis is 45% and is greater in those with colonic than ileal disease, particularly in individuals with rectal involvement [6].

The cumulative probability of major abdominal surgery in CD at 5, 10, and 20 years after diagnosis is 38, 48, and 58%, respectively [7]. Small bowel location of disease, upper gastrointestinal involvement or ileocolonic disease, current smoking, male gender, and penetrating disease behavior predict eventual need for surgery. In two large cohorts, the risk of major abdominal surgery in CD was unchanged over time [7, 8] whereas other cohorts demonstrated that increasing use and earlier institution of effective treatments were associated with decrease in rates of surgery [9, 10]. Genetic variants such as *NOD2* may also impact the risk of ileal fibrostenosis [11, 12]. Perianal disease has been variably associated with need for abdominal surgery, but may increase the risk of stricturing and penetrating complications in CD.

## Diagnosis

### History and Physical Examination

A comprehensive history in patients with CD should include assessment of symptoms related to the disease, extraintestinal manifestations, eliciting features that may differentiate it from other causes, solicitation of symptoms related to potential complications of disease, and ascertainment of risk factors for adverse events related to therapy, in addition to effect of disease on work status, functioning, and quality of life. History taking should also include family history and assessment of potential environmental risk factors contributing to disease risk or natural history. Cigarette smoking is an important and modifiable risk factor for CD associated with a more aggressive disease course and should be noted. Enteric infections and NSAIDs are sometimes triggers for relapses in patients with established CD. Information should be obtained on antibiotic use, as antibiotic-associated *Clostridium difficile* infection has been associated with disease flares. Depression and anxiety are common and may influence quality of life and social functioning [13, 14]. A comprehensive history should also include evaluation for complications of CD, including perianal manifestations, symptoms suggestive of occlusive small bowel or colonic disease, and presence of extraintestinal manifestations. In children, information on growth and development is essential as in some patients, small bowel CD may present with failure to thrive or growth retardation, including delay of puberty, as the only manifestation.

There are several well-established indices for the assessment of disease activity in CD. The Crohn's disease activity index (CDAI) was developed by Best *et al.* [15] and consists of eight factors, each weighted differently, namely number of liquid stools, abdominal pain, general well-being, presence of extraintestinal complications, need for antidiarrheals or narcotics, presence of abdominal mass on physical examination, hematocrit, and percentage deviation from standard weight. The CDAI, although widely used in clinical trials, correlates poorly with objective markers of inflammation and is cumbersome to incorporate in routine clinical practice. A CDAI below 150 suggests clinical remission whereas values between 220 and 450 indicate moderate

Table 2.3 The Crohn's disease activity index (CDAI): a CDAI <150 indicates remission, 150–220 indicates mild disease, 220–450 indicates moderate disease, and >450 indicates severe disease.

| Parameter | Weighting factor |
| --- | --- |
| Number of liquid or soft stools each day | ×2 |
| Abdominal pain (graded from 0 to 3 on severity) | ×5 |
| General well-being [0 (well) to 4 (terrible)] | ×7 |
| Presence of complications[a] | ×20 |
| Use of antidiarrheals | ×30 |
| Presence of abdominal mass (0, none; 2, questionable; 5, definite) | ×10 |
| Hematocrit <47% in mean or 42% in women | ×6 |
| Percentage deviation from standard weight | ×1 |

[a] 1 point each for arthralgia or arthritis; iritis or uveitis; erythema nodosum, pyoderma gangrenosum, or aphthous ulcers; anal fissures, fistulae or abscesses; other fistulae; fever.
*Source:* Adapted from Best *et al.* 1976 [15]. Reproduced with permission of Elsevier.

disease activity (Table 2.3). Values in between represent mild disease and values above 450 represent severe disease activity. Other indices such as the Harvey–Bradshaw index correlate well with CDAI and may be easier to incorporate into clinical practice.

Abdominal examination may reveal tenderness in the right lower quadrant, the most common site of involvement. In patients with an inflammatory phlegmon or ileocecal abscess, a right lower quadrant mass may be palpable. Features of weight loss, anemia (pallor), and nutritional deficiencies may be visible on general physical examination. Full examination may also reveal the presence of extraintestinal manifestations. A thorough perianal examination is essential to identify perianal complications such as abscess, fistulae, skin tags, or anal stricture. Physical examination should also include ascertaining whether extraintestinal manifestations such as erythema nodosum, pyoderma gangrenosum, arthritis, or ocular manifestations are present. (See Chapter 4.)

### Laboratory Investigations

Anemia is a common laboratory abnormality in CD and may be multifactorial from deficiency of iron, vitamin $B_{12}$, or folic acid, chronic gastrointestinal blood loss, or anemia of chronic disease. A baseline evaluation should include a complete blood count, metabolic profile, including liver and renal functions, and assessment for nutritional deficiencies. Iron and ferritin levels should be obtained at baseline but ferritin, an acute-phase protein, may be falsely elevated in active inflammation. Vitamin $B_{12}$ deficiency is common in patients with ileal involvement. Many patients are deficient in vitamin D. In patients with prolonged active disease or severe disease, a low serum albumin is seen. Urinalysis may reveal the presence of calcium oxalate crystals or red blood cells in the setting of nephrolithiasis. Stool examination will reveal the presence of fecal leukocytes and is non-specific. Microbiologic evaluation should be performed to rule out infectious causes of diarrhea due to enteric pathogens, ova and parasites, and *C. difficile*.

Measurements of erythrocyte sedimentation rate (ESR) and C-reactive protein are useful for initial diagnosis and monitoring of patients with CD. Between 70 and 100% of patients have an elevated C-reactive protein; a smaller number demonstrate an elevation in ESR [16, 17]. C-reactive protein is also useful in predicting relapse, and as a biomarker to predict response to therapy [18]. Fecal markers of inflammation such as calprotectin and lactoferrin may be useful to rule out intestinal inflammation in patients with a low index of suspicion for inflammatory bowel disease (IBD), but have less of a role in small bowel CD as they are less frequently elevated compared with colonic disease. As CD often presents with diarrhea alone without overt bleeding mimicking functional bowel disease, fecal calprotectin may be a useful screening test, particularly in children and normal values below 50 μg g$^{-1}$ of stool may make it possible to avoid the need for a colonoscopy [19, 20]. Fecal calprotectin levels also correlate with endoscopy disease activity and are more sensitive than symptom-based indices such as the CDAI. Fecal lactoferrin has a similar utility [21].

### Serologic Markers

Several serologic markers are elevated in CD; the range that correlates with CD is wider than that seen in UC. Most biomarkers identified in CD are directed against microbial targets. The most common of these is the anti-*Saccharomyces cerevisiae* antibody (ASCA IgA and IgG) directed against the cell wall of the yeast *Saccharomyces*, first reported by Main *et al.* in 1988 [22]. Elevated ASCA levels are present in 29–69% of patients with CD and 0–29% of patients with UC, but may also be seen in 0–23% of patients with other gastrointestinal diseases, limiting their utility to establish a diagnosis or screen at-risk individuals [23]. The anti-OmpC antibody against the OmpC transport protein of *Escherichia coli* is seen in 24–55% of patients with CD and in a much smaller number of patients with other gastrointestinal diseases (5–12%). The anti-CBir1 antibody, directed again bacterial flagellin, is identified in 50–56% of patients with CD. Less commonly found antibodies are antiglycan antibodies against the cell wall [anti-laminaribioside carbohydrate IgG antibodies (ALCA), anti-chitobioside carbohydrate IgA antibodies (ACCA), and anti-mannobioside carbohydrate IgG antibodies (AMCA)] [24]. These may have utility in patients who are negative for ASCA [23]. Although these antibodies have good specificity in differentiating CD from UC (77–100%), the sensitivity and negative predictive values remain low, particularly in screening patients with gastrointestinal symptoms, limiting their utility in diagnosis. These antibodies may precede the diagnosis of IBD [25]. Higher titers of antibodies and the presence of multiple antimicrobial antibodies are associated with more aggressive disease behavior, increasing risk of penetrating and stricturing complications and surgery [26–28].

### Endoscopy

Lower gastrointestinal endoscopy is essential to establish the diagnosis of CD, differentiate it from UC, define the extent and severity of disease, assess response to treatment, and screen for dysplasia. Rectal involvement is seen in about half of patients with colonic CD compared with the nearly universal (>95%) presence of rectal inflammation in patients with UC. In contrast to the contiguous pattern of inflammation in UC, that in CD tends to be discontinuous with segments of normal0appearing bowel (skip areas) intervening between segments of involved colon. Inflammation presents as focal ulceration or aphthous ulcers, which are small, discrete ulcers surrounded by a thin rim of erythematous tissue. Other forms of ulcers seen in CD include serpiginous or linear ulcers, punched-out or deep ulcers, cobblestoning, which represents nodular mucosa intersected by crisscrossing linear ulcerations, and large stellate confluent ulcers (Figure 2.3).

Several scoring systems have been developed to quantify endoscopic disease activity, the two most common being the Crohn's disease endoscopic index of severity (CDEIS) (Table 2.4) [29] and the simple endoscopic score in Crohn's disease (SES-CD) [30]. The SES-CD is easier to incorporate into clinical practice and consists of sums of scores from each of the ileal and colonic segments for ulcer size, proportion of ulcerative surface, affected surface, and presence of luminal narrowing. Similar endoscopic changes can be identified in other sites of involvement. A subgroup of patients with CD may have focal enhanced gastritis on gastric biopsy in the absence of *H. pylori* infection, and this finding can be used to establish a diagnosis of CD when the diagnosis is otherwise uncertain [31, 32]. A separate endoscopic score has been developed to quantify severity of endoscopic recurrence following ileocecal resection, ranging from i0 to i4 [33] (Table 2.5). A score of i2 or greater indicates significant endoscopic recurrence.

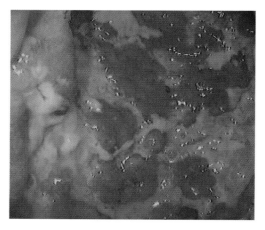

**Figure 2.3** Endoscopic appearance of colonic Crohn's disease with wide ulcerations, edema, and intervening areas of normal mucosa.

**Table 2.5** Rutgeerts classification of post-operative recurrence in Crohn's disease.

| Score | Endoscopic appearance |
|---|---|
| 0 | Normal |
| 1 | <5 apthous ulcers |
| 2 | >5 aphthous ulcers, normal mucosa between ulcers, or lesions confined to the anastomosis |
| 3 | Diffuse ileitis |
| 4 | Diffuse inflammation with large ulcers, nodularity, and stenosis |

**Table 2.4** Table for calculation of Crohn's disease endoscopic index of severity (CDEIS).

| | Rectum | Sigmoid and left colon | Transverse colon | Right colon | Ileum | |
|---|---|---|---|---|---|---|
| Deep ulceration: if present, score 12; if absent, score 0 | | | | | | Total 1 |
| Superficial ulceration: if present, score 12; if absent, score 0 | | | | | | Total 2 |
| Surface involved by the disease measured in cm | | | | | | Total 3 |
| Ulcerated surface measured in cm | | | | | | Total 4 |
| Total 1 + Total 2 + Total 3 + Total 4 = | | | | | | A |
| Number (*n*) of segments totally or partially explored (1–5) = | | | | | | *n* |
| Total A divided by *n* = | | | | | | B |
| Ulcerated stenosis: if present anywhere, score 3; if absent, score 0 = | | | | | | C |
| Non-ulcerated stenosis: if present anywhere, score 3; if absent, score 0 = | | | | | | D |
| TOTAL B + C + D = | | | | | | |

*Source:* Adapted from Mary and Modigliani 1989 [29]. Reproduced with permission of BMJ Publishing Group.

Wireless capsule endoscopy has greater utility in CD than UC because of the frequent need to assess the small intestine beyond the reach of most endoscopes. In a meta-analysis of nine studies including patients with suspected CD, the yield of capsule endoscopy was superior to ileocolonoscopy (63% versus 23%), computed tomography enterography (CTE) (30%), or magnetic resonance imaging (22%) [34]. Capsule endoscopy can also be used to monitor for mucosal healing in small bowel CD, but has a higher rate of capsule retention in established disease. In patients with a suspected small bowel stricture contributing to their symptoms, an alternative cross-sectional modality to rule out obstructive lesions should be performed prior to performing a video capsule endoscopy.

### Histology

Histologic findings in CD, in parallel with the endoscopic appearance, are usually focal. Crypt architectural irregularity and chronic inflammation are focal and patchiness is common. The inflammation is transmural, although this is usually not identifiable on endoscopic biopsies. Lymphoid aggregates are common. The pathognomonic feature in CD is the presence of non-caseating granulomas; however, this is seen in only 30% of patients (Figure 2.4). Granulomas may also be seen in spared areas of mucosa, lymph nodes, mesentery, peritoneum, and liver. Similar to UC, inflammatory pseudopolyps may be found. Pyloric gland metaplasia is seen in 2–27% of ileal biopsies in CD and in ileal resections and is uncommon in UC.

### Imaging Studies

Cross-sectional imaging studies are useful to diagnose extent of involvement and complications in CD and are frequently complementary to lower gastrointestinal endoscopy. Air contrast barium studies, single- or double-contrast barium studies, and barium small bowel follow through may have a role in specific clinical situations but are now used infrequently unless newer preferred modalities are not available. Abdominal ultrasound with contrast is helpful in assessing wall thickness, strictures, and postoperative recurrence but is dependent on operator expertise and body habitus [35–37].

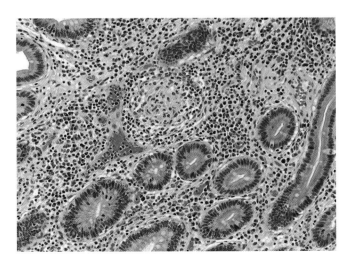

**Figure 2.4** Histologic appearance of the small bowel in Crohn's disease demonstrating a single discrete non-necrotizing granuloma. *Source*: Reproduced with permission of Vikram Deshpande MD.

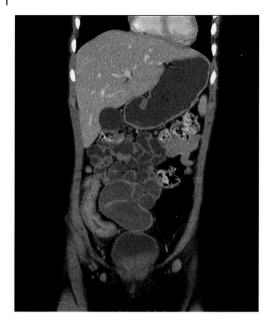

**Figure 2.5** Active terminal ileal Crohn's disease on CTE demonstrating wall thickening, mucosal hyperenhancement, and mesenteric inflammation.

Computed tomography enterography (CTE) achieves distension of the lumen of the small bowel through the administration of a large volume of neutral oral contrast, commonly 0.1% low-density barium sulfate. Intravenous contrast is also administered in conjunction. Findings indicative of CD include bowel wall thickening, mural enhancement and stratification, and the "comb sign," which refers to increased mesenteric vascularity and engorgement of the vasa recta [38] (Figure 2.5). The sensitivity of CTE in detecting CD is approximately 90%. In addition, cross-sectional imaging is very useful to detect fistulae, abscesses, and strictures. Dynamic changes identifiable on CTE can be used to monitor response to treatment and as a marker of early treatment response [39]. However, an abdominal CT scan has low utility in diagnosis of perianal disease and pelvic complications as the imaging studies are often not extended deep into the pelvis and have low resolution in the region.

Patients with CD are young and often undergo multiple imaging studies during their lifetime [40]. Consequently, magnetic resonance enterography (MRE), which uses a similar technique as in the CT scan but utilizes MR imaging instead, is increasingly utilized to avoid cumulative exposure to ionizing radiation. The relevant findings on an MRE are very similar to that from a CTE and comparative studies have suggested similar or superior ability of MR imaging to distinguish active inflammatory disease from chronic fibrostenotic disease [41–43]. In addition, MR imaging is also the most useful imaging modality for the detection and characterization of the perianal fistulae [38].

The differential diagnosis for CD is discussed in conjunction with UC in Chapter 3, but many features that can be used to distinguish the two are summarized in Table 2.2.

## Case Studies and Multiple Choice Questions

1  Amy is a 19-year-old college student who is seeking a second opinion regarding a recent diagnosis of IBD. She had presented to her primary care physician with symptoms of weight loss, generalized abdominal pain, and diarrhea. A colonoscopy performed at diagnosis revealed multiple scattered aphthous ulcerations throughout the colon, beginning in the sigmoid colon and extending to the cecum. The ileum appeared macroscopically normal. Biopsies demonstrated crypt abscesses, architectural irregularity, and focal active inflammation throughout the affected colon. Which of the following statements is true about Amy's diagnosis?

A  Her diagnosis is ulcerative colitis because of involvement restricted to the colon and not involving the ileum.

B  Her diagnosis is ulcerative colitis because the absence of granulomas rules out a diagnosis of Crohn's disease.

C  Her diagnosis is Crohn's colitis because of rectal sparing and presence of aphthous ulcerations throughout the colon.

D  Her diagnosis is infectious colitis because of the presence of crypt abscesses and focal active inflammation.

2  Which potential future clinical course is likely for Amy?

A  Because of its isolated involvement of the colon, Amy has a higher likelihood of needing surgery over the next 10 years.

B  Her likelihood of developing stricturing or penetrating complications is less than it would have been if she also had ileal involvement.

C  She is more likely to carry a polymorphism at the NOD2 locus.

D  She has a 70% likelihood of developing ileal ulcerations over the next 5 years.

3  Which of the following serologic patterns are most likely if Amy is tested?

A  Elevated ASCA and negative pANCA (perinuclear antineutrophil cytoplasmic antibody).

B  Negative ASCA and elevated pANCA.

C  Elevated OmpC and negative ASCA and pANCA.

D  Elevated tissue transglutaminase and anti-gliadin antibodies.

4  Which of the following risk factors have not been associated with a more progressive and disabling course of Crohn's disease?

A  Age less than 40 years.

B  Perianal involvement.

C  Need for steroids at diagnosis.

D  Coexisting extraintestinal manifestations.

## References

1 Cosnes, J., Cattan, S., Blain, A., *et al.* (2002) Long-term evolution of disease behavior of Crohn's disease. *Inflammatory Bowel Diseases*, **8**(4), 244–250.

2 Lazarev, M., Huang, C., Bitton, A., *et al.* (2013) Relationship between proximal Crohn's disease location and disease behavior and surgery: a cross-sectional study of the IBD Genetics Consortium. *American Journal of Gastroenterology*, **108**(1), 106–112.

3 Cosnes, J., Gower-Rousseau, C., Seksik, P., and Cortot, A. (2011) Epidemiology and natural history of inflammatory bowel diseases. *Gastroenterology*, **140**(6), 1785–1794.

4 Thia, K.T., Sandborn, W.J., Harmsen, W.S., *et al.* (2010) Risk factors associated with progression to intestinal complications of Crohn's disease in a population-based cohort. *Gastroenterology*, **139**(4), 1147–1155.

5 Louis, E., Collard, A., Oger, A.F., *et al.* (2001) Behaviour of Crohn's disease according to the Vienna classification: changing pattern over the course of the disease. *Gut*, **49**(6), 777–782.

6 Schwartz, D.A., Loftus, E.V., Jr., Tremaine, W.J., *et al.* (2002) The natural history of fistulizing Crohn's disease in Olmsted County, Minnesota. *Gastroenterology*, **122**(4), 875–880.

7 Peyrin-Biroulet, L., Harmsen, W.S., Tremaine, W.J., *et al.* (2012) Surgery in a population-based cohort of Crohn's disease from Olmsted County, Minnesota (1970–2004). *American Journal of Gastroenterology*, **107**(11), 1693–1701.

8 Cosnes, J., Nion-Larmurier, I., Beaugerie, L., *et al.* (2005) Impact of the increasing use of immunosuppressants in Crohn's disease on the need for intestinal surgery. *Gut*, **54**(2), 237–241.

9 Lakatos, P.L., Golovics, P.A., David, G., *et al.* (2012) Has there been a change in the natural history of Crohn's disease? Surgical rates and medical management in a population-based inception cohort from Western Hungary between 1977–2009. *American Journal of Gastroenterology*, **107**(4), 579–588.

10 Ramadas, A.V., Gunesh, S., Thomas, G.A., *et al.* (2010) Natural history of Crohn's disease in a population-based cohort from Cardiff (1986–2003): a study of changes in medical treatment and surgical resection rates. *Gut*, **59**(9), 1200–1206.

11 Abreu, M.T., Taylor, K.D., Lin, Y.C., *et al.* (2002) Mutations in *NOD2* are associated with fibrostenosing disease in patients with Crohn's disease. *Gastroenterology*, **123**(3), 679–688.

12 Adler, J., Rangwalla, S.C., Dwamena, B.A., and Higgins, P.D. (2011) The prognostic power of the *NOD2* genotype for complicated Crohn's disease: a meta-analysis. *American Journal of Gastroenterology*, **106**(4), 699–712.

13 Ananthakrishnan, A.N., Gainer, V.S., Perez, R.G., *et al.* (2013) Psychiatric

co-morbidity is associated with increased risk of surgery in Crohn's disease. *Alimentary Pharmacology & Therapeutics*, **37**(4), 445–454.

14  Bitton, A., Dobkin, P.L., Edwardes, M.D., *et al.* (2008) Predicting relapse in Crohn's disease: a biopsychosocial model. *Gut*, **57**(10), 1386–1392.

15  Best, W.R., Becktel, J.M., Singleton, J.W., and Kern, F., Jr. (1976) Development of a Crohn's disease activity index. National Cooperative Crohn's Disease Study. *Gastroenterology*, **70**(3), 439–444.

16  Vermeire, S., Van Assche, G., and Rutgeerts, P. (2006) Laboratory markers in IBD: useful, magic, or unnecessary toys? *Gut*, **55**(3), 426–431.

17  Vermeire, S., Van Assche, G., and Rutgeerts, P. (2005) The role of C-reactive protein as an inflammatory marker in gastrointestinal diseases. *Nature Clinical Practice Gastroenterology & Hepatology*, **2**(12), 580–586.

18  Hibi, T., Sakuraba, A., Watanabe, M., *et al.* (2014) C-reactive protein is an indicator of serum infliximab level in predicting loss of response in patients with Crohn's disease. *Journal of Gastroenterology*, **49**(2), 254–262.

19  Schoepfer, A.M., Beglinger, C., Straumann, A., *et al.* (2010) Fecal calprotectin correlates more closely with the Simple Endoscopic Score for Crohn's disease (SES-CD) than CRP, blood leukocytes, and the CDAI. *American Journal of Gastroenterology*, **105**(1), 162–169.

20  Sipponen, T., Karkkainen, P., Savilahti, E., *et al.* (2008) Correlation of faecal calprotectin and lactoferrin with an endoscopic score for Crohn's disease and histological findings. *Alimentary Pharmacology & Therapeutics*, **28**(10), 1221–1229.

21  Sipponen, T., Savilahti, E., Kolho, K.L., *et al.* (2008) Crohn's disease activity assessed by fecal calprotectin and lactoferrin: correlation with Crohn's disease activity index and endoscopic findings. *Inflammatory Bowel Diseases*, **14**(1), 40–46.

22  Main, J., McKenzie, H., Yeaman, G.R., *et al.* (1998) Antibody to *Saccharomyces cerevisiae* (bakers' yeast) in Crohn's disease. *British Medical Journal (Clinical Research Edition)*, **297**(6656), 1105–1106.

23  Prideaux, L., De Cruz, P., Ng, S.C., and Kamm, M.A. (2012) Serological antibodies in inflammatory bowel disease: a systematic review. *Inflammatory Bowel Diseases*, **18**(7), 1340–1355.

24  Ferrante, M., Henckaerts, L., Joossens, M., *et al.* (2007) New serological markers in inflammatory bowel disease are associated with complicated disease behaviour. *Gut*, **56**(10), 1394–1403.

25  Israeli, E., Grotto, I., Gilburd, B., *et al.* (2005) Anti-*Saccharomyces cerevisiae* and antineutrophil cytoplasmic antibodies as predictors of inflammatory bowel disease. *Gut*, **54**(9), 1232–1236.

26  Lichtenstein, G.R., Targan, S.R., Dubinsky, M.C., *et al.* (2011) Combination of genetic and quantitative serological immune markers are associated with complicated Crohn's disease behavior. *Inflammatory Bowel Diseases*, **17**(12), 2488–2496.

27  Dubinsky, M.C., Lin, Y.C., Dutridge, D., *et al.* (2006) Serum immune responses predict rapid disease progression among children with Crohn's disease: immune responses predict disease progression. *American Journal of Gastroenterology*, **101**(2), 360–367.

28  Desir, B., Amre, D.K., Lu, S.E., *et al.* (2004) Utility of serum antibodies in determining clinical course in pediatric Crohn's disease. *Clinical Gastroenterology and Hepatology*, **2**(2), 139–146.

29  Mary, J.Y. and Modigliani, R. (1989) Development and validation of an endoscopic index of the severity for Crohn's disease: a prospective multicentre study. Groupe d'Etudes Thérapeutiques

des Affections Inflammatoires du Tube Digestif (GETAID). *Gut*, **30**(7), 983–989.

30  Daperno, M., D'Haens, G., Van Assche, G., *et al.* (2004) Development and validation of a new, simplified endoscopic activity score for Crohn's disease: the SES-CD. *Gastrointestinal Endoscopy*, **60**(4), 505–512.

31  Parente, F., Cucino, C., Bollani, S., *et al.* (2000) Focal gastric inflammatory infiltrates in inflammatory bowel diseases: prevalence, immunohistochemical characteristics, and diagnostic role. *American Journal of Gastroenterology*, **95**(3), 705–711.

32  Oberhuber, G., Puspok, A., Oesterreicher, C., *et al.* (1997) Focally enhanced gastritis: a frequent type of gastritis in patients with Crohn's disease. *Gastroenterology*, **112**(3), 698–706.

33  Rutgeerts, P., Geboes, K., Vantrappen, G., *et al.* (1984) Natural history of recurrent Crohn's disease at the ileocolonic anastomosis after curative surgery. *Gut*, **25**(6), 665–672.

34  Triester, S.L., Leighton, J.A., Leontiadis, G.I., *et al.* (2006) A meta-analysis of the yield of capsule endoscopy compared to other diagnostic modalities in patients with non-stricturing small bowel Crohn's disease. *American Journal of Gastroenterology*, **101**(5), 954–964.

35  Dong, J., Wang, H., Zhao, J., *et al.* (2014) Ultrasound as a diagnostic tool in detecting active Crohn's disease: a meta-analysis of prospective studies. *European Radiology*, **24**(1), 26–33.

36  Paredes, J.M., Ripolles, T., Cortes, X., *et al.* (2013) Contrast-enhanced ultrasonography: usefulness in the assessment of postoperative recurrence of Crohn's disease. *Journal of Crohn's & Colitis*, **7**(3), 192–201.

37  Calabrese, E., La Seta, F., Buccellato, A., *et al.* (2005) Crohn's disease: a comparative prospective study of transabdominal ultrasonography, small intestine contrast ultrasonography, and small bowel enema. *Inflammatory Bowel Diseases*, **11**(2), 139–145.

38  Grand, D.J., Harris, A., and Loftus, E.V., Jr. (2012) Imaging for luminal disease and complications: CT enterography, MR enterography, small-bowel follow-through, and ultrasound. *Gastroenterology Clinics of North America*, **41**(2), 497–512.

39  Bruining, D.H., Loftus, E.V., Jr., Ehman, E.C., *et al.* (2011) Computed tomography enterography detects intestinal wall changes and effects of treatment in patients with Crohn's disease. *Clinical Gastroenterology and Hepatology*, **9**(8), 679–683.e1.

40  Peloquin, J.M., Pardi, D.S., Sandborn, W.J., *et al.* (2008) Diagnostic ionizing radiation exposure in a population-based cohort of patients with inflammatory bowel disease. *American Journal of Gastroenterology*, **103**(8), 2015–2022.

41  Rimola, J., Rodriguez, S., Garcia-Bosch, O., *et al.* (2009) Magnetic resonance for assessment of disease activity and severity in ileocolonic Crohn's disease. *Gut*, **58**(8), 1113–1120.

42  Rimola, J., Ordas, I., Rodriguez, S., and Panes, J. (2010) Colonic Crohn's disease: value of magnetic resonance colonography for detection and quantification of disease activity. *Abdominal Imaging*, **35**(4), 422–427.

43  Rimola, J., Ordas, I., Rodriguez, S., *et al.* (2012) Imaging indexes of activity and severity for Crohn's disease: current status and future trends. *Abdominal Imaging*, **37**(6), 958–966.

44  Beaugerie, L., Seksik, P., Nion-Larmurier, I., *et al.* (2006) Predictors of Crohn's disease. *Gastroenterology*, **130**(3), 650–656.

## Answers to Questions

1   Answer: **C**. Although the ileum remains the most common site affected, up to 20% of patients with Crohn's disease will have isolated inflammation in the colon. The presence of typical aphthous ulcerations and rectal lend further support to a diagnosis of Crohn's disease. Granulomas, although supportive of a diagnosis of Crohn's disease, are present in only 20–30% of patients and their absence does not rule out a diagnosis of Crohn's disease.

2   Answer: **B**. Patients with colonic disease tend to remain inflammatory or uncomplicated for many years whereas those with ileal locations progress to complications faster and more frequently [27]. NOD2 mutations have been associated with ileal and fibrostenosing phenotype of Crohn's disease and do not occur at an increased frequency in those with isolated Crohn's colitis. In contrast to disease behavior, disease location tends to be stable; extension to the small bowel occurs in fewer than 20% of patients with initial isolated colonic disease 10 years after diagnosis [29].

3   Answer: **A**. The most common serologic pattern in Crohn's disease is elevated ASCA levels along with a negative pANCA. The inverse (pANCA elevation with negative ASCA) is more typical in ulcerative colitis. Anti-OmpC antibodies are found in a subset of patients with Crohn's disease but at a lower frequency than ASCA and so would not be the most common serologic pattern. Patients with Crohn's disease are not at a higher risk of developing celiac disease.

4   Answer: **D**. In a large prospective French cohort of 1188 patients with Crohn's disease followed for 5 years, the requirement for steroids at diagnosis [odds ratio (OR) 3.1, 95% confidence interval (CI) 2.2–4.4], age below 40 years (OR 2.1, 95% CI 1.3–3.6), and perianal involvement (OR 1.8, 95% CI 1.2–2.8) were associated with disabling disease with a positive predictive value of 91 and 93% with the presence of two or three factors, respectively [44].

# 3

# Clinical Features and Diagnosis of Ulcerative Colitis

## Clinical Take Home Messages

- Ulcerative colitis is characterized by diffuse inflammation beginning in the rectum and extending contiguously proximally.
- Approximately one-quarter of patients have colitis involving the entire colon ("pancolitis") at presentation. For patients with distal disease at diagnosis, disease extension may occur in up to one-third.
- Approximately 10–20% of patients with UC require colectomy during the course of their disease.
- Serologic (C-reactive protein, erythrocyte sedimentation rate) and fecal (calprotectin) markers of inflammation are useful for monitoring disease activity, assessing response to treatment, and predicting risk of relapse.
- Colonoscopic and histologic examination reveals a contiguous pattern of transmucosal and submucosal inflammation characterized by frequent crypt abscesses, crypt architectural irregularities, and mucin depletion. Histologic activity may predict risk of relapse and subsequent development of colorectal neoplasia.

The hallmark of ulcerative colitis (UC) is superficial and diffuse inflammation, usually beginning in the rectum and extending proximally, involving contiguous segments of the colon. While UC is restricted to the colon, approximately 10–20% of patients with pancolitis may have mild ileal inflammation termed backwash ileitis [1]. Some patients with isolated distal disease may have a patch of endoscopic inflammation in the cecal base and peri-appendiceal area termed "cecal patch." This does not have specific clinical significance and the natural history of such patients resembles that of others with distal disease.

The clinical features and natural history of UC generally correlate with the extent of inflammation. According to the Montreal classification, extent is categorized as proctitis if the inflammation is restricted to the rectum. Extension to the sigmoid colon, 15–20 cm beyond the anal verge, is termed proctosigmoiditis. Left-sided colitis and pancolitis refer to inflammation up to and beyond the splenic flexure, respectively (Table 3.1). The Paris modification of the Montreal classification for pediatric UC further separated those with extension beyond the splenic flexure into extensive colitis, referring to extension up to the hepatic flexure,

*Inflammatory Bowel Diseases: A Clinician's Guide*, First Edition. Ashwin N. Ananthakrishnan, Ramnik J. Xavier, and Daniel K. Podolsky.
© 2017 John Wiley & Sons Ltd. Published 2017 by John Wiley & Sons Ltd.

Table 3.1 Montreal classification of extent and severity of ulcerative colitis.

| | | |
|---|---|---|
| Extent | E1 | Involvement limited to the rectum |
| | E2 | Involvement limited to the colorectal distal to the splenic flexure |
| | E3 | Involvement extending proximal to the splenic flexure |
| Severity | S0 (remission) | Asymptomatic |
| | S1 (mild) | ≤4 stools per day (with or without blood), no systemic features, normal inflammatory markers |
| | S2 (moderate) | >4 stools per day but no systemic toxicity |
| | S3 (severe) | >6 stools per day, pulse rate of 90 $min^{-1}$, temperature >37.5 °C, hemoglobin <10.5 g per 100 ml, ESR >30 mm $h^{-1}$ |

or pancolitis, when the inflammation extends proximal to the hepatic flexure. At the time of diagnosis, approximately one-third of patients have disease limited to the rectum, another one-third have extension to the splenic flexure, and the disease is proximal to the splenic flexure in another one-third of patients. Approximately one-quarter of patients have pancolitis involving the entire colon. One-third of patients with initial diagnosis of distal disease can develop proximal extension; regression of pancolitis is uncommon.

## Clinical Features

The hallmark of UC is diarrhea and rectal bleeding. In most patients, the onset is insidious, and in some, it can be traced to cessation of or a reduction in their cigarette consumption. Rectal bleeding varies in amount and is usually mixed with mucous pus. In patients with isolated proctitis, this may be the dominant symptom without any increase in stool frequency. Symptoms of urgency and tenesmus and a sense of incomplete evacuation are also common in patients with proctitis or rectal involvement. Often patients report multiple bowel movements clustered together, or inability to distinguish between gas, blood, and stool. Patients with proctitis or proctosigmoiditis may actually have constipated bowel movements because

of delayed colonic transit. Severe abdominal pain is unusual in mild to moderate UC, but left-sided colicky abdominal pain preceding bowel movements is common.

Patients with more extensive colitis commonly experience diarrhea and overt bleeding. Owing to involvement beginning in the rectum, such patients can also have the distal symptoms described above. Systemic features are more common in patients with extensive colitis and include weight loss and anemia. A small subset of patients may present with fulminant colitis or toxic megacolon, usually in the context of extensive colitis. Such patients have prominent fever, severe abdominal pain, distension, and abdominal tenderness with peritoneal signs on examination. Similarly to Crohn's disease (CD), patients may present with extraintestinal manifestations at their first presentation with the colitis. Such manifestations are more common in those with extensive colitis.

Several scoring systems have been developed to stratify UC by severity. One of the most commonly used scales was developed by Truelove and Witts for the initial landmark trial establishing the efficacy of cortisone in the treatment of UC [2]. The criteria defined mild, severe, and fulminant disease based on the clinical parameters of stool frequency, presence of blood in the stool, temperature, pulse, and two laboratory parameters – erythrocyte sedimentation rate (ESR) and hematocrit (Table 3.2). Patients

Table 3.2 Truelove–Witts classification of severity of ulcerative colitis.

| Criterion | Mild | Severe | Fulminant |
|---|---|---|---|
| Stools (no. per day) | <4 | >6 | >10 |
| Blood in stool | Intermittent | Frequent | Continuous |
| Temperature (°C) | Normal | >37.5 | >37.5 |
| Pulse (beats min$^{-1}$) | Normal | >90 | >90 |
| Hematocrit (%) | Normal | <75% | Transfusion |
| ESR (mm h$^{-1}$) | <30 | >30 | >30 |

with mild disease have fewer than four bowel movements per day, only intermittent blood in their stool, and no systemic features. In contrast, patients with severe disease have in excess of six bowel movements per day, frequent rectal bleeding, fever, tachycardia, anemia, and elevated inflammation markers. Nocturnal symptoms are common in patients with severe disease. Sudden cessation of bowel movements accompanied by increasing abdominal pain or distension should trigger suspicion for toxic megacolon.

## Disease Course and Natural History

Most patients with UC have flares alternating with periods of remission. A small proportion may have progressive or persistent symptoms. Relapses are usually difficult to predict but may sometimes have discernible triggers such as non-adherence to medical therapy, non-steroidal agent use, or enteric infections. The severity of relapses is often difficult to predict. In a large cohort in Copenhagen County, Denmark, disease activity within the first year of diagnosis was fulminant in 9%, moderate to high in 71%, and low in only 20% of patients [3]. Within the first year of diagnosis, 50% of patients with UC experienced a relapse [4]. In a 10-year follow-up of the IBSEN cohort in Norway, an initial severe flare followed by

mild intermittent flares was the most common pattern of disease activity, occurring in 55% of patients [5]. A chronic intermittent symptom course was the next most common disease pattern, occurring in one-third of the patients (37%). Chronic continuous symptoms occurred infrequently (6%), as did an initial mild presentation followed by escalating severity (1%). The cumulative rates of colectomy at 1, 5, and 10 years after diagnosis were 4, 8, and 10%, respectively. The likelihood of requiring surgery was higher in those with extensive colitis (19%) than those with left-sided colitis (8%) or proctitis (5%). Nearly half of the colectomies were carried out within the first 2 years after diagnosis.

## Diagnosis

The diagnosis of UC is based on a combination of clinical, endoscopic, and histologic features. In about 10% of patients, it is difficult to distinguish between UC and CD, despite complete history, physical examination, and laboratory and endoscopic evaluation, and is termed inflammatory bowel disease-unclassified (IBDU) or indeterminate colitis. A subset of such patients develop more typical features of CD on follow-up, but many patients remain indeterminate throughout their course.

### History and Physical Examination

A comprehensive history at the time of diagnosis of suspected UC should target evaluation of severity of disease, differential diagnoses that may mimic UC, extraintestinal manifestations, and potential environmental influences. History should be obtained on frequency and character of bowel movements, amount and frequency of bleeding, and proportion of bowel movements with visible blood. Abdominal pain, cramping, tenesmus, urgency, and sense of incomplete evacuation may be helpful in determining severity of distal disease. Significant diarrhea alone in the absence of rectal bleeding is infrequent in UC. Information should also be obtained on the presence and frequency of nocturnal bowel movements and clustering of bowel movements. Systemic features such as weight loss are helpful in estimating severity of disease. Potential environmental triggers of IBD or clues for alternative diagnoses include history of recent travel, use of non-steroidal anti-inflammatory drugs (NSAIDs), current and past smoking, diet, personal history of other autoimmune diseases, and family history of IBD which may be seen in approximately 10% of patients. Information should also be obtained on clinical factors that may determine increased risk of complications associated with potential therapies, including susceptibility to infections, cardiac disease, coexisting demyelinating disease, or other rheumatologic conditions. A reproductive history including plans for pregnancy in the future should be noted.

General physical examination will reveal the presence of pallor in the case of significant anemia, and jaundice with coexisting primary sclerosing cholangitis (PSC). Physical examination may otherwise be normal except for mild left-sided abdominal tenderness. Rebound or guarding on physical examination is uncommon with uncomplicated UC and should raise suspicion for transmural complications, such as toxic megacolon. Bowel sounds are usually normal but may be diminished or absent in patients with toxic megacolon. Presence of anal skin tags or perianal fistulae should raise suspicion for CD. Erythema nodosum lesions may accompany UC and present as small nodules on the lower extremities, primarily on the shin. Arthritis presents as erythema, swelling, and tenderness of the inflamed joints. (See Chapter 4.)

### Laboratory Investigations

All patients with suspected UC should have a complete blood count and metabolic panel including renal and liver function tests. Isolated elevation of alkaline phosphatase may be the only clue to the presence of coexisting PSC. Elevated platelet count, ESR, and C-reactive protein (CRP), anemia, and low serum albumin are common in active disease and correlate generally with disease severity. CRP elevation is seen in 50–60% of patients with active UC [6]. In a prospective pediatric cohort study including 451 children with UC, ESR thresholds of 23, 23–29, 30–37, and >37 mm h$^{-1}$ were used to distinguish quiescent, mild, moderate, and severe disease activity, respectively [7]. However, both CRP and ESR may be normal in 34% of those with mild and in 5–10% of those with moderate-to-severe disease. Some patients may demonstrate an elevation in only one of the inflammatory markers. Consequently, it is useful to obtain both at diagnosis, and then to use one for serial monitoring of disease activity [7]. All patients with suspected UC should undergo stool testing for enteric pathogens, *Clostridium difficile* infection, ova, and parasites. Fecal leukocytes are sometimes elevated in patients, reflecting inflammatory etiology of their diarrhea. Quantitative fecal hemoglobin has been proposed by some as a measure of disease severity but is not widely used.

As noted in Chapter 2, the granulocyte-derived calcium binding protein calprotectin is a promising stool marker of gut inflammation. In a prospective study of 228 patients with UC and 52 healthy controls, endoscopic disease activity demonstrated superior correlation with fecal calprotectin ($r = 0.821$) compared with clinical indices ($r = 0.682$), CRP ($r = 0.556$), or hemoglobin ($r = -0.388$) [8]. Fecal calprotectin was also useful in differentiating grades of endoscopic activity. At a threshold of 57 µg g$^{-1}$, it had a sensitivity of 91% and specificity of 90% in detecting endoscopically active disease defined as a Baron index of ≥2 [8]. Fecal calprotectin levels 3 months after initial therapy in newly diagnosed UC was predictive of disease course over 3 years of follow-up although the accuracy was modest [9]. Rapidity of decrease of fecal calprotectin may predict clinical remission with infliximab use [10] and colectomy in hospitalized patients [11].

**Serologic Markers**

Serologic markers can be useful in the evaluation of patients with suspected UC. Patients with UC are most likely to have a pattern characterized by an elevation in perinuclear antineutrophil cytoplasmic antibody (pANCA) and negative anti-*Saccharomyces cerevisiae* antibody (ASCA) levels whereas patients with CD have the inverse pattern of elevated ASCA with undetectable pANCA. The exact antigen of pANCA is unclear but it may target the nuclear DNA-bound protein H1 [12]. Three-quarters (50–80%) of patients with UC have elevated pANCA. A systematic review concluded that pANCA positivity had high specificity (98%) and positive predictive value (98%) in distinguishing patients with IBD from healthy individuals, but low sensitivity (17%) and negative predictive value (16%) [13]. The combination of ASCA+/pANCA− had a sensitivity of 52–64% in

distinguishing CD from UC, but the sensitivity was lower for colonic CD (30–38%) and the positive predictive value in both settings was at best fair (76–95%) [13]. One setting where there is clinical utility for serologic testing is in patients with IBDU. A total of 64% of patients who were ASCA−/pANCA+ in this clinical scenario declared themselves as having UC over long-term follow-up whereas 80% of patients who were ASCA+/pANCA− developed CD [14]. Patients who were seronegative for both were likely to remain seronegative and remained IBDU. There are limited data suggesting prognostic value for serologic testing in UC. The presence of antimicrobial antibodies, particularly those associated with CD such as the ASCA [15] or antiflagellin antibody (anti-CBir1), was associated with increased risk of pouchitis following total proctocolectomy and ileoanal anastomosis [16] and postoperative fistulae whereas high levels of pANCA were predictive of chronic pouchitis [17].

**Endoscopy**

Lower gastrointestinal endoscopy is essential for the diagnosis of UC. Inflammation almost always (>95%) begins in the rectum and extends proximally in a contiguous fashion. The characteristic endoscopic findings are erythema, friability, loss of normal colonic vascular markings, and granularity. Spontaneous hemorrhage or deep ulcerations are uncommon and indicate severe disease. It is often useful to establish extent of inflammation at diagnosis as this may determine the need for oral systemic therapy and subsequent surveillance intervals. However, in patients with severe disease at presentation, it is advisable not to proceed with a full colonoscopy owing to increased risk of perforation. As noted above, some patients with distal disease may have an isolated patch of inflammation in the cecum or periappendiceal region. The clinical significance of this is unclear, but it does not appear to indicate a more severe course of disease or a diagnosis of CD. Exudates of mucous or mucopus are common. Up to 20% of patients with pancolitis may have superficial ileal erythema, termed backwash ileitis. However, deep ileal ulcers are uncommon and should raise suspicion for CD. With institution of treatment and healing of the mucosa, inflammatory pseudopolyps may develop, representing heaped up areas of granulation tissue. These are rarely symptomatic and usually have no neoplastic potential, although patients with

extensive pseudopolyposis may have a modest increase in risk of colon cancer. However, the presence of these pseudopolyps sometimes makes it challenging to distinguish visible adenomatous from non-dysplastic inflammatory lesions.

Several endoscopic scores have been developed to quantify severity of endoscopic inflammation. One of the most widely used is the Mayo endoscopic score, which stratifies patients into normal, mild, moderate, or severe disease (Figure 3.1) [18]. A score of

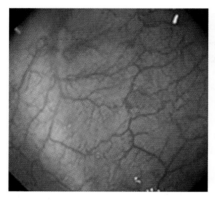

0 Normal or inactive disease

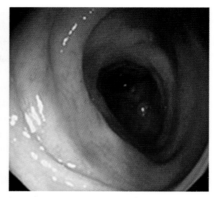

1 Mild disease (erythema, decreased vascular pattern, mild friability)

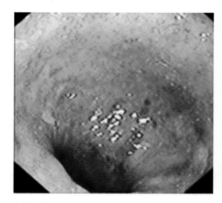

2 Moderate disease (marked erythema, absent vascular pattern, friability, erosions)

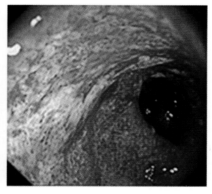

3 Severe disease (spontaneous bleeding, ulcerations)

**Figure 3.1**  Mayo endoscopic score for assessment of disease activity in ulcerative colitis. *Source:* Pineton de Chambrun *et al.* 2010 [18]. Reproduced with permission of Nature Publishing Group.

0 represents normal or inactive disease; a score of 1 is characterized by erythema, decreased vascular pattern, and mild friability; a score of 2 indicates marked erythema, friability, and presence of ulcerations; and a score of 3 represents severe disease and is characterized by spontaneous bleeding and ulceration. A more recently validated risk score is the ulcerative colitis endoscopic index of severity (UCEIS) [19], a composite score incorporating a scale ranging from 1 to 3 points for vascular pattern, from 1 to 4 points for bleeding, and from 1 to 4 points for erosions and ulcerations (Table 3.3). The UCEIS correlates well with overall assessment of severity ($r = 0.93$) and inflammatory markers [20], and is reliable and valid in clinical practice [21]. An upper gastrointestinal endoscopy is usually not essential except in the presence of symptoms suggesting distinct upper gastrointestinal disease. Even in patients with UC, mild macroscopic or histologic inflammation may be seen in the stomach in up to 40% of children and does not indicate CD [22].

**Table 3.3** Ulcerative colitis endoscopic index of severity.

*Vascular pattern*
  0 = Normal
  1 = Patchy obliteration
  2 = Obliterated

*Bleeding*
  0 = None
  1 = Mucosal
  2 = Luminal mild
  3 = Luminal moderate or severe

*Erosions and ulcers*
  0 = None
  1 = Erosions
  2 = Superficial ulcer
  3 = Deep ulcer

Score the worst-affected segment.
*Source:* Adapted from Travis *et al.* 2012 [19]. Reproduced with permission of BMJ Publishing Group.

### Histology

The hallmark of UC regarding histology is demonstration of chronic inflammation and architectural distortion on histology (Figure 3.2). The primary aim with histology is to distinguish chronic UC from acute

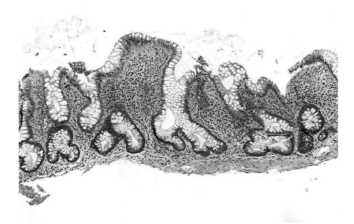

**Figure 3.2** Biopsy from an individual with ulcerative colitis. Colonic mucosa with histologic evidence of chronic colitis. Note the marked crypt architectural distortion including crypt branching. An increased number of lymphocytes and plasma cells are present throughout the lamina propria.

Table 3.4 Histologic findings in ulcerative colitis and acute self-limited colitides.

|  | Ulcerative colitis | Acute self-limited colitis |
| --- | --- | --- |
| Distorted crypt architecture | 32[a] | 0 |
| Mixed lamina propria inflammation | 15[a] | 0 |
| Villous surface | 22[a] | 0 |
| Crypt atrophy | 16[a] | 0 |
| Basal lymphoid aggregates | 12[a] | 0 |
| Surface erosions | 21[a] | 4 |
| Superficial isolated giant cell | 3 | 7 |
| Basal isolated giant cell | 6 | 1 |
| Polymorphonuclear cells in the surface epithelium | 19 | 9 |

[a]$p < 0.05$.
*Source:* Adapted from Surawicz and Belic 1984 [23]. Reproduced with permission of Elsevier.

self-limited colitis [23] (Table 3.4). Biopsy from the rectum indicating disease involvement from the rectum can be useful in differentiating UC from CD [23]. Biopsies from the ileum may detect backwash ileitis. Crypt architectural irregularity is continuous, as is chronic inflammation that decreases proximally. The inflammation is superficial but sometimes extends into the submucosa. Crypt abscesses are common, and goblet cell mucin depletion in biopsies may be pronounced. Granulomas are usually not seen in UC [24]. Certain histologic features may have prognostic significance. In a prospective study of 82 patients with chronic quiescent ulcerative colitis, the presence of acute inflammatory infiltrate, crypt abscesses, and mucin depletion was associated with increased rates of relapse. However, chronic inflammatory cell infiltrate and architectural irregularities had no prognostic significance [25]. Histologic activity may also correlate with subsequent risk of colorectal cancer.

### Imaging Studies

Cross-sectional imaging studies are needed only infrequently in UC. Typical findings in patients with longstanding and extensive UC on barium contrast exam include a foreshortened and featureless colon without distinct haustrations. A plain abdominal film in patients hospitalized with acute severe colitis is useful to investigate the presence of toxic megacolon or detect actual perforation by the presence of free intra-abdominal air. In patients where the distinction between CD and UC is not clear, cross-sectional abdominal imaging with computed tomography enterography (CTE) or magnetic resonance enterography (MRE) is helpful. In small studies, MR colography correlated well with severe endoscopic disease in the sigmoid colon and rectum [26]. The presence of relative contrast enhancement, edema, enlarged lymphoma nodes, and the "comb" sign (increased mesenteric vascularity) were independent predictors of disease activity in UC. A combined segmental index identified endoscopic inflammation with a sensitivity of 87% and specificity of 88% [27].

## Differential Diagnosis (UC and CD)

Several conditions can mimic IBD. In a patient presenting with diarrhea, particularly chronic diarrhea, the differential diagnosis is wide. The first step is to establish the inflammatory nature of the diarrhea. This can be determined by assessment for fecal leukocytes (inexpensive but insensitive), other fecal markers such as calprotectin or lactoferrin, and serologic markers such as CRP (Figure 3.3). Weight loss, nocturnal symptoms, and rectal bleeding are all more common in IBD and are rarely seen with functional gastrointestinal disease. Distal colitis may sometimes present with constipation rather than diarrhea and mimic rectal bleeding from hemorrhoids or anal fissures. NSAID-related enteritis or colitis is sometimes difficult to distinguish from underlying IBD, as both clinical features and endoscopic changes may mimic ulceration in CD. However, chronicity of inflammation often favors IBD over acute NSAID-related colitis or enteritis.

An acute presentation of IBD can sometimes be difficult to distinguish from infectious causes, as markers of inflammation will be elevated in both. On initial presentation of IBD, it is important to rule out enteric pathogens both as an alternative diagnosis and as a trigger for IBD. This includes stool testing for *Salmonella, Shigella, Escherichia coli* O157:H7, *Campylobacter,* and *Giardia* and, if indicated, serologic testing for amebiasis. Infectious colitis is usually self-limited and resolves within a few days. Endoscopically, infectious colitis may resemble IBD. Amebiasis can present with punched-out ulcers in the ileocecal region resembling CD. *C. difficile,* an important cause of healthcare-associated diarrhea, is increasingly prevalent in the community and may resemble IBD endoscopically, including the presence of mucopus resembling pseudomembranes.

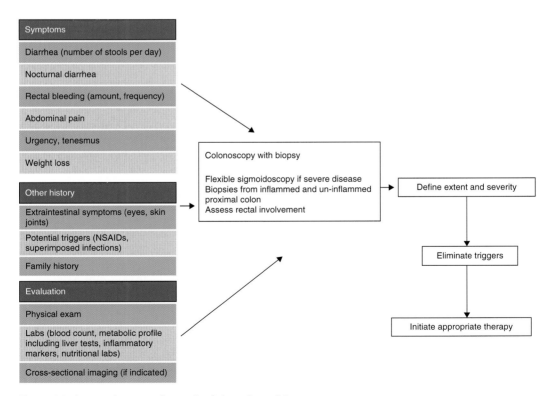

**Figure 3.3** Approach to new diagnosis of ulcerative colitis.

Sexual transmission of pathogens such as *Chlamydia, Herpes, Neisseria gonorrhoeae,* and *Treponema pallidum* may cause proctitis resembling IBD. Solitary rectal ulcer syndrome can also present as isolated proctitis with rectal bleeding, urgency, and mucous discharge. Patients often report a history of straining. Endoscopically, circumferential or semi-circumferential ulceration is seen in the distal rectum, just proximal to the anorectal junction. Histologically, mucosal prolapse and fibromuscular hyperplasia in the lamina propria are found. Cytomegalovirus (CMV) colitis can mimic IBD in immunosuppressed patients. Superimposed CMV infection, often in the setting of immunosuppressed therapy for the underlying UC, can be responsible for a flair or failure to improve on therapy. Mucosal biopsy, particularly from the right colon, can reveal large intranuclear inclusion indicative of infection.

With the increasing incidence of IBD in regions with a high prevalence of tuberculosis (TB), it may be challenging to differentiate intestinal TB from CD. Similarly to CD, intestinal TB has a predilection for the ileum and cecum and may present with diarrhea, abdominal pain, weight loss, and right lower quadrant mass [28]. Systemic symptoms of fevers and night sweats are more common with intestinal TB than CD and concomitant symptoms of pulmonary disease may be present. Endoscopic features are similar; both can manifest as strictures, fistulae, and ulcerations. However, perianal disease is uncommon with TB. The relatively infrequent identification of tubercle bacilli on Gram staining or on polymerase chain reaction (PCR) on biopsies from patients with suspected intestinal TB makes the distinction all the more challenging. Histologically, TB demonstrates caseating granulomas, more than 10 granulomas from biopsies, increased submucosal inflammation, and epithelioid histiocytes. However, up to one-quarter of patients eventually

diagnosed with CD initially receive a therapeutic trial with anti-TB therapy where lack of response and subsequent response to steroids point towards a diagnosis of CD.

Acute right lower quadrant pain may be difficult to differentiate from acute appendicitis. There is often a preceding history of chronic diarrhea or intermittent abdominal pain in patients with CD, but an acute presentation is seen in some patients where the distinction is sometimes apparent only in the operating room. A ruptured appendix with surrounding inflammation may make the site of origin of the penetrating complication difficult to identify. *Yersinia* enteritis can present as acute right lower quadrant inflammation and pain, with the diagnosis made by stool culture. Celiac disease is common in the North American population and presents as diarrhea, abdominal cramping, weight loss, anemia, and low vitamin D, which can occasionally mimic CD. Although celiac disease is not more common among patients with CD, patients with celiac disease are more likely to develop either CD or UC. Hence a high index of suspicion for celiac disease and appropriate serologic testing are important.

Other rare causes of diarrhea that are sometimes difficult to distinguish clinically from CD include Whipple's disease, Behcet's disease, and intestinal lymphoma. Whipple's disease presents with diarrhea, weight loss, anemia, and arthritis with laboratory evidence of malabsorption. The diagnosis is made by histopathologic evidence of periodic acid–Schiff-positive inclusions within macrophages. Intestinal lymphoma can present with diarrhea, and systemic features such as fevers, night sweats, and weight loss and an intestinal mass. Behcet's disease presents with a combination of oral and genital ulcers and uveitis and may be difficult to distinguish from CD [29].

Microscopic colitis (collagenous colitis and lymphocytic colitis) presents as watery secretory diarrhea in older patients and is diagnosed histologically by the presence of a thickened subepithelial collagen layer in the colon or lymphocytic infiltration. Endoscopically, microscopic colitis appears normal or mild erythema is present. Diverticulitis and ischemic colitis are sometimes difficult to distinguish from UC, particularly in older patients. Endoscopically, ischemic colitis is often restricted to watershed areas with involvement of the splenic flexure. Pancolonic involvement or involvement of the rectum is unusual with ischemic colitis as the rectum has extensive collateral circulation. Systemic vasculitis, particularly polyarteritis nodosa and Henoch–Schönlein purpura, can also present with diarrhea, abdominal pain, and rectal bleeding, but is often accompanied by other extraintestinal symptoms.

Differentiating underlying IBD from an alternative cause can be particularly challenging in the setting of colonic diversion. This may be seen in patients with a Hartmann's pouch with either a temporary or permanent diversion for perianal CD or after subtotal colectomy for UC prior to ileoanal anastomosis construction. The endoscopic findings of so-called diversion colitis and underlying IBD are similar, and a therapeutic trial of antibiotics or short-chain fatty acids may be required to establish the former diagnosis empirically.

## Case Studies and Multiple Choice Questions

1  Mary is a 45-year-old woman with a diagnosis of left-sided ulcerative colitis established on colonoscopy 10 years prior to her consultation with you. Which of the following is a statement of clinical course for a patient with Mary's history?

A Proximal extension is nearly universal in patients with an initial diagnosis of distal colitis and Mary is highly likely to develop pancolitis over the next 10 years.

B Up to one-third of patients with distal disease may expect proximal extension of their disease.

C She has a less than 10% risk of progression to proximal colitis over the natural history of her disease.

2  After your first consultation, you perform a colonoscopy in Mary. This reveals inflammation from the rectum to the splenic flexure, normal transverse colon, and ascending colon, with mild inflammation seen around the appendiceal orifice. Which of the following is true about this "cecal patch"?

A Patients with distal colitis and a cecal patch have a natural history that is similar to those with pancolitis and should be managed as such.

B The presence of a cecal patch has not been associated with more aggressive disease behavior in patients with distal disease.

C The presence of a cecal patch indicates a diagnosis of Crohn's disease as it reflects "skip lesions."

D The presence of a cecal patch is associated with an increased risk of colorectal cancer.

3  Mary's 18-year-old son presents to you with ongoing diarrhea and generalized abdominal cramping for 3 months. Given his family history and suggestive symptoms, your recommend a colonoscopy. However, he is reluctant to undergo the procedure unless he absolutely needs it and inquires about the availability of non-invasive methods to establish a diagnosis of ulcerative colitis. Which of the following tests would be associated with the highest negative predictive value for an underlying diagnosis of inflammatory bowel disease?

A Normal C-reactive protein.

B Normal hemoglobin and albumin.

C Normal fecal calprotectin.

D Normal IBD-7 serology.

4  Which of the following histologic features is uncommon in patients with chronic ulcerative colitis?

A Crypt architectural distortion.

B Focal active inflammation.

C Mucin depletion and surface erosions.

D Presence of crypt abscesses.

# References

1  Heuschen, U.A., Hinz, U., Allemeyer, E.H., *et al.* (2001) Backwash ileitis is strongly associated with colorectal carcinoma in ulcerative colitis. *Gastroenterology*, **120**(4), 841–847.

2  Truelove, S.C. and Witts, L.J. (1954) Cortisone in ulcerative colitis; preliminary report on a therapeutic trial. *British Medical Journal*, **ii**(4884), 375–378.

3  Langholz, E., Munkholm, P., Nielsen, O.H., *et al.* (1991) Incidence and prevalence of ulcerative colitis in Copenhagen county from 1962 to 1987. *Scandinavian Journal of Gastroenterology*, **26**(12), 1247–1256.

4  Moum, B., Ekbom, A., Vatn, M.H., *et al.* (1997) Clinical course during the 1st year after diagnosis in ulcerative colitis and Crohn's disease. Results of a large, prospective population-based study in southeastern Norway, 1990–93. *Scandinavian Journal of Gastroenterology*, **32**(10), 1005–1012.

5  Solberg, I.C., Lygren, I., Jahnsen, J., *et al.* (2009) Clinical course during the first 10 years of ulcerative colitis: results from a population-based inception cohort (IBSEN Study). *Scandinavian Journal of Gastroenterology*, **44**(4), 431–440.

6  Vermeire, S., Van Assche, G., and Rutgeerts, P. (2006) Laboratory markers in IBD: useful, magic, or unnecessary toys? *Gut*, **55**(3), 426–431.

7  Turner, D., Mack, D.R., Hyams, J., *et al.* (2011) C-reactive protein (CRP), erythrocyte sedimentation rate (ESR) or both? A systematic evaluation in pediatric ulcerative colitis. *Journal of Crohn's & Colitis*, **5**(5), 423–429.

8  Schoepfer, A.M., Beglinger, C., Straumann, A., *et al.* (2013) Fecal calprotectin more accurately reflects endoscopic activity of ulcerative colitis than the Lichtiger Index, C-reactive protein, platelets, hemoglobin, and blood leukocytes. *Inflammatory Bowel Diseases*, **19**(2), 332–341.

9  Lasson, A., Simren, M., Stotzer, P.O., *et al.* (2013) Fecal calprotectin levels predict the clinical course in patients with new onset of ulcerative colitis. *Inflammatory Bowel Diseases*, **19**(3), 576–581.

10 De Vos, M., Dewit, O., D'Haens, G., *et al.* (2012) Fast and sharp decrease in calprotectin predicts remission by infliximab in anti-TNF naive patients with ulcerative colitis. *Journal of Crohn's & Colitis*, **6**(5), 557–562.

11 Travis, S., Satsangi, J., and Lemann, M. (2011) Predicting the need for colectomy in severe ulcerative colitis: a critical appraisal of clinical parameters and currently available biomarkers. *Gut*, **60**(1), 3–9.

12 Eggena, M., Cohavy, O., Parseghian, M.H., *et al.* (2000) Identification of histone H1 as a cognate antigen of the ulcerative colitis-associated marker antibody pANCA. *Journal of Autoimmunity*, **14**(1), 83–97.

13 Prideaux, L., De Cruz, P., Ng, S.C., and Kamm, M.A. (2012) Serological antibodies in inflammatory bowel disease: a systematic review. *Inflammatory Bowel Diseases*, **18**(7), 1340–1355.

14  Joossens, S., Reinisch, W., Vermeire, S., *et al.* (2002) The value of serologic markers in indeterminate colitis: a prospective follow-up study. *Gastroenterology*, **122**(5), 1242–1247.

15  Dendrinos, K.G., Becker, J.M., Stucchi, A.F., *et al.* (2006) Anti-*Saccharomyces cerevisiae* antibodies are associated with the development of postoperative fistulas following ileal pouch-anal anastomosis. *Journal of Gastrointestinal Surgery*, **10**(7), 1060–1064.

16  Fleshner, P., Ippoliti, A., Dubinsky, M., *et al.* (2008) Both preoperative perinuclear antineutrophil cytoplasmic antibody and anti-CBir1 expression in ulcerative colitis patients influence pouchitis development after ileal pouch–anal anastomosis. *Clinical Gastroenterology and Hepatology*, **6**(5), 561–568.

17  Fleshner, P.R., Vasiliauskas, E.A., Kam, L.Y., *et al.* (2001) High level perinuclear antineutrophil cytoplasmic antibody (pANCA) in ulcerative colitis patients before colectomy predicts the development of chronic pouchitis after ileal pouch–anal anastomosis. *Gut*, **49**(5), 671–677.

18  Pineton de Chambrun, G., Peyrin-Biroulet, L., Lémann, M., and Colombel, J.F. (2010) Clinical implications of mucosal healing for the management of IBD. *Nature Reviews Gastroenterology & Hepatology*, **7**(1), 15–29.

19  Travis, S.P., Schnell, D., Krzeski, P., *et al.* (2012) Developing an instrument to assess the endoscopic severity of ulcerative colitis: the Ulcerative Colitis Endoscopic Index of Severity (UCEIS). *Gut*, **61**(4), 535–542.

20  Samuel, S., Bruining, D.H., Loftus, E.V., Jr., *et al.* (2013) Validation of the ulcerative colitis colonoscopic index of severity and its correlation with disease activity measures. *Clinical Gastroenterology and Hepatology*, **11**(1), 49–54.e1.

21  Travis, S.P., Schnell, D., Krzeski, P., *et al.* (2013) Reliability and initial validation of the Ulcerative Colitis Endoscopic Index of Severity. *Gastroenterology*, **145**(5), 987–995.

22  Kovacs, M., Muller, K.E., Arato, A., *et al.* (2012) Diagnostic yield of upper endoscopy in paediatric patients with Crohn's disease and ulcerative colitis. Subanalysis of the HUPIR registry. *Journal of Crohn's & Colitis*, **6**(1), 86–94.

23  Surawicz, C.M. and Belic, L. (1984) Rectal biopsy helps to distinguish acute self-limited colitis from idiopathic inflammatory bowel disease. *Gastroenterology*, **86**(1), 104–113.

24  Magro, F., Langner, C., Driessen, A., *et al.* (2013) European consensus on the histopathology of inflammatory bowel disease. *Journal of Crohn's & Colitis*, **7**(10), 827–851.

25  Riley, S.A., Mani, V., Goodman, M.J., *et al.* (1991) Microscopic activity in ulcerative colitis: what does it mean? *Gut*, **32**(2), 174–178.

26  Savoye-Collet, C., Roset, J.B., Koning, E., *et al.* (2012) Magnetic resonance colonography in severe attacks of ulcerative colitis. *European Radiology*, **22**(9), 1963–1971.

27  Ordás, I., Rimola, J., García-Bosch, O., *et al.* (2013) Diagnostic accuracy of magnetic resonance colonography for the evaluation of disease activity and severity in ulcerative colitis: a prospective study. *Gut*, **62**(11), 1566–1572.

28  Makharia, G.K., Srivastava, S., Das, P., *et al.* (2010) Clinical, endoscopic, and histological differentiations between Crohn's disease and intestinal tuberculosis. *American Journal of Gastroenterology*, **105**(3), 642–651.

29  Lee, S.K., Kim, B.K., Kim, T.I., and Kim, W.H. (2009) Differential diagnosis of intestinal Behcet's disease and Crohn's disease by colonoscopic findings. *Endoscopy*, **41**(1), 9–16.

30  Sinclair, T.S., Brunt, P.W., and Mowat, N.A. (1983) Nonspecific proctocolitis in northeastern Scotland: a community study. *Gastroenterology*, **85**(1), 1–11.

31  Byeon, J.S., Yang, S.K., Myung, S.J., *et al.* (2005) Clinical course of distal ulcerative colitis in relation to appendiceal orifice inflammation status. *Inflammatory Bowel Diseases*, **11**(4), 366–371.

## Answers to Questions

1 Answer: **B**. In a prospective cohort, up to one-third of patients with distal colitis develop proximal extension at 10 years [30].

2 Answer: **B**. A cecal patch may be seen in 3–10% of patients with distal colitis and is not associated with an increased risk for aggressive disease behavior or risk of colorectal cancer in patients with distal ulcerative colitis [31].

3 Answer: **C**. Both CRP and ESR may be normal in up to 34% of those with mild and 5–10% of those with moderate-to-severe disease. Hence normal values in those with mild symptoms cannot be used to rule out UC as an underlying diagnosis. In a prospective study of 228 patients with UC and 52 healthy controls, endoscopic disease activity demonstrated superior correlation with fecal calprotectin ($r = 0.821$) compared with clinical indices ($r = 0.682$), CRP ($r = 0.556$), or hemoglobin ($r = -0.388$) [8]. An IBD-7 serology test has suboptimal sensitivity and specificity to establish a diagnosis without supportive evidence and should not be used to rule in or rule out a diagnosis of IBD.

4 Answer: **B**. Focal active inflammation in the gastrointestinal tract is more commonly seen in Crohn's disease than ulcerative colitis, where the inflammation tends to be contiguous.

# 4

# Extraintestinal Manifestations of Inflammatory Bowel Diseases

---

## Clinical Take Home Messages

- Extraintestinal manifestations (EIMs) occur in one-third of patients with inflammatory bowel disease (IBD) and variably may precede, occur concurrently with, or follow the diagnosis of IBD.
- Among EIMs, peripheral and axial arthritis are the most common. The activity of peripheral arthritis usually parallels underlying luminal disease activity whereas axial arthropathy is usually independent of bowel symptoms.
- Metabolic bone disease is common in IBD. Patients with a history of vertebral fractures, males older than 50 years of age, postmenopausal women, those on chronic corticosteroid therapy, or those with hypogonadism should undergo screening for osteoporosis with a dual-energy X-ray absorptiometry (DEXA) scan.
- Primary sclerosing cholangitis (PSC) may occur in 2–4% of patients with IBD and is associated with increased risk of colorectal cancer. Consequently, such patients should undergo an annual surveillance colonoscopy exam. Pericholangitis, a form of inflammation that may represent the mildest form of PSC, may be present in up to 80% of patients.
- IBD is associated with increased risk for venous thromboembolism, particularly in the setting of hospitalization.
- Skin manifestations include erythema nodosum, which may presage a flare of disease activity, and pyoderma gangrenosum, a potentially devastating complication without a consistent association with disease activity.
- Ocular manifestations including uveitis, scleritis, and episcleritis are less common but may be severe, and are usually found in association with active disease.

---

Extraintestinal manifestations (EIMs) are common and occur in one-third of patients with inflammatory bowel disease (IBD) (Table 4.1). They may precede, occur concurrently with, or follow the diagnosis of IBD. Some EIMs parallel luminal symptoms whereas others may be independent of the natural history of bowel disease. EIMs are usually more common in ulcerative colitis (UC) than Crohn's disease (CD), and among patients with CD, more common in those with colonic involvement.

*Inflammatory Bowel Diseases: A Clinician's Guide*, First Edition. Ashwin N. Ananthakrishnan, Ramnik J. Xavier, and Daniel K. Podolsky.
© 2017 John Wiley & Sons Ltd. Published 2017 by John Wiley & Sons Ltd.

Table 4.1 Major extraintestinal manifestations of inflammatory bowel diseases.

| Organ system | Manifestation |
|---|---|
| Dermatologic | Erythema nodosum, pyoderma gangrenosum, necrotizing vasculitis, psoriasiform lesions, cutaneous Crohn's disease, aphthous ulcers (oral) |
| Musculoskeletal | Arthralgia, arthropathy (axial and appendicular), osteoporosis, avascular necrosis |
| Hepatobiliary | Primary sclerosing cholangitis, autoimmune hepatitis, pericholangitis, granulomatous hepatitis, gallstones, fatty liver |
| Renal | Nephrolithiasis (calcium oxalate) |
| Ophthalmologic | Scleritis, episcleritis, uveitis, retinal vascular occlusive disease |
| Hematologic | Iron deficiency anemia, anemia of chronic disease, vitamin $B_{12}$ deficiency, venous thromboembolism |

## Arthritis and Arthropathy

The most common EIM in IBD is arthropathy, occurring in 5–20% of patients. It can be classified into that involving the axial skeleton and that affecting the appendicular (peripheral) skeleton. Peripheral arthropathy can be further subdivided into type 1 and type 2 depending on the pattern of joint involvement. Type I peripheral arthropathy affects 4–8% of patients with IBD, usually involves the large joints (elbows, knees), is pauciarticular (less than five joints), and is asymmetric [1]. It frequently parallels activity of underlying bowel disease. Type 2 peripheral arthropathy is usually symmetrical and polyarticular, involving the small joints of the upper limbs. The activity of type 2 peripheral arthropathy may be independent of bowel symptoms. Peripheral arthropathy can be associated with other EIMs, in particular erythema nodosum (type 1) and uveitis (both types) [1, 2]. Genetically, type 1 arthropathy has been associated with HLA-DRB1*0103 in 33%, DRB*35 in 30%, and HLA-B27 in 26% of patients [3]. In contrast, type 2 is associated primarily with HLA-B*44 [3]. Arthritic flares in IBD tend to be non-erosive and non-deforming. Treatment is often challenging if acetaminophen is not sufficient as a pain reliever as anti-inflammatory agents such as non-steroidal anti-inflammatory drugs (NSAIDs) may themselves trigger luminal disease flares. COX-2-selective agents may be safe for use in the short term without triggering bowel symptoms. Antitumor necrosis factor-α (anti-TNF) biologic agents have very good efficacy in the management of peripheral arthritis associated with IBD. Sulfasalazine (owing to the antiarthritic effect of the sulfapyridine moiety) and methotrexate are also good options for the treatment of IBD-associated arthropathy.

Sacroiliitis, a limited form of axial arthritis, is seen in 2–32% of patients with IBD but may be detected incidentally on radiologic imaging in some patients [3] (Figure 4.1). It manifests as low back pain, associated morning stiffness, and improvement with physical activity. It is frequently independent of underlying bowel disease, although it parallels activity of bowel disease in some [3]. It may also precede the development of IBD. Between 5 and 10% of patients with ankylosing spondylitis (AS) have definite IBD, although a larger proportion have subclinical intestinal inflammation with findings not sufficient to establish a diagnosis of IBD definitively [4]. Most patients with IBD-associated AS are HLA-B27 positive. The natural history of AS is usually independent of the underlying bowel disease and may be progressively

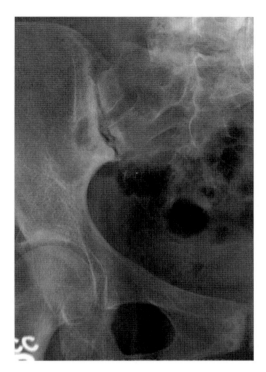

**Figure 4.1** Plain radiograph of right sacroiliac joint in a patient with ulcerative colitis and sacroileitis.

deforming, leading to a stooped posture and loss of lumbar lordosis. Radiographic changes include squaring of the vertebrae, development of syndesmophytes, and appearance of "bamboo spine" due to bridging of the intervertebral discs. As with peripheral arthritis, management of AS in IBD is challenging owing to its progressive nature and the inability of many to tolerate long-term NSAID use, which can exacerbate the underlying IBD. Physical therapy can help maintain flexibility of the spine. Selective COX-2 inhibitors and intermittent use of narcotics may alleviate the pain. Recent placebo-controlled trials have examined the efficacy of anti-TNF agents in AS. A systematic review of nine trials, two using infliximab, five using etanercept, and two using adalimumab, demonstrated a threefold greater response rate with anti-TNF treatment compared with placebo at

12 weeks [5]. Functional scores were also improved at 12 weeks, suggesting that such agents may be an option for treatment of IBD-associated AS. However, it is important to note that etanercept is not effective in the management of underlying IBD; consequently, other anti-TNF biologics may be superior choices to treat both bowel and joint disease.

## Metabolic Bone Disease

Metabolic bone disease is common and occurs in as many as half of patients with IBD. In particular, CD is associated with an increased risk of osteoporosis of the lumbar spine and femur [6]. Risk factors contributing to impaired bone mineral density include disease-specific factors such as malabsorption (of calcium and vitamin D), malnutrition (poor oral intake due to symptoms of active disease, ongoing inflammatory burden), reduced physical activity, vitamin D deficiency, corticosteroid exposure, and small bowel resection resulting in reduced capacity for absorption. Patients with ileal disease and those with underlying PSC are particularly vulnerable owing to malabsorption of fat-soluble vitamins. Inflammatory cytokines such as TNF-$\alpha$ can also activate osteoclasts, leading to enhanced bone resorption. Disease-independent factors such as age, post-menopausal status, low body mass index, and smoking also contribute to impaired bone density. Whether the higher frequency of impaired bone density translates to increased risk of fractures is unclear, as the literature in this area is inconsistent. Some studies suggested an increase in fracture risk in patients with IBD [7–9] whereas others found no such association [10–13]. The American Gastroenterological Association guidelines recommend screening with dual-energy X-ray absorptiometry (DEXA) in patients with IBD with one or more of the following risk factors: history of

**Table 4.2** Recommendations for screening and treatment of osteoporosis in patients with inflammatory bowel diseases.

*Screening with a DEXA scan is recommended for all patients with ≥1 risk factor. In patients with normal values, repeat testing should be performed every 2–3 years*

 History of vertebral fractures

 Postmenopausal women

 Males older than 50 years of age

 Chronic corticosteroid therapy

 Hypogonadism

*Treatment of osteoporosis*

*Pharmacologic therapy*

 Calcium and vitamin D supplementation

 Bisphosphonates

 Calcitonin

 Recombinant parathyroid hormone (PTH)

*Non-pharmacologic therapy*

 Weight-bearing exercise

 Quitting smoking

 Limited alcohol consumption

 Minimizing corticosteroid use

vertebral fractures, males older than 50 years of age, postmenopausal women, those on chronic corticosteroid therapy, or with hypogonadism [14]. Treatment of osteoporosis and osteopenia in IBD is similar to that in the general population [15] (Table 4.2).

## Cutaneous Manifestations

The two most common cutaneous manifestations of IBD are erythema nodosum (EN) (Figure 4.2) and pyoderma gangrenosum (PG) (Figure 4.3). PG occurs in 1–5% of patients with UC and less frequently in CD, where it is associated with colonic involvement. It usually begins as an ulcer with a necrotic base on the lower extremities, which can become large, deep, and destructive, healing with permanent scarring. The activity of PG parallels underlying bowel disease in half of the patients. It may also occur

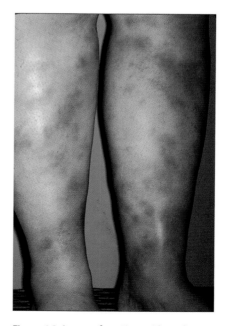

**Figure 4.2** Image of a patient with erythema nodosum. *Source:* William D. James, University of Pennsylvania.

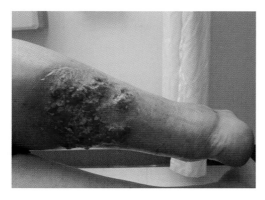

**Figure 4.3** Pyoderma gangrenosum in a patient with inflammatory bowel disease.

frequently at the sites of previous trauma, including the peristomal region. Diagnosis is established clinically but may be supported by biopsy from the ulcer edge, demonstrating folliculitis and dense neutrophilic infiltration.

Management of pyoderma begins with local wound care and topical or intralesional corticosteroids for mild disease. In patients with severe or refractory disease, systemic treatment with steroids, immunomodulators, cyclosporine, or anti-TNF biologic therapy may be necessary. Anti-TNF biologics appear to be very effective in the management of this complication [16]. PG can occur in sites of trauma, especially after abdominal surgery or as peristomal lesions. Treatment of such pyoderma is similar to that at other sites. PG may recur when revision of the site of a stoma is undertaken.

EN is seen more commonly in CD, presenting as erythematous nodules on the lower extremity, usually over the anterior surface of the tibia. Its activity usually parallels underlying bowel disease and is sometimes manifest before obvious recurrent gastrointestinal symptoms. EN responds to treatment of the bowel disease.

Despite anti-TNF therapy itself being an effective treatment for idiopathic psoriasis, some patients with IBD on anti-TNF therapy experience paradoxical immune activation resulting in psoriasiform lesions [17, 18]. The underlying mechanism for this paradoxical effect is unclear but has been hypothesized to relate to the unregulated production of interferon-$\alpha$ by plasmacytoid dendritic cells that infiltrate the skin early during the development of psoriasis [19]. Anti-TNF-induced psoriasiform lesions are more common in women (70%); the palmoplantar area (43%) and scalp (42%) are the most common sites of distribution [17]. In a case series of 120 published cases, 41% were noted to respond to topical treatment but 43% required withdrawal of the offending agent for resolution of the lesion. Recurrence of the lesion was noted in half of the patients who retried a second anti-TNF agent [17].

## Hepatobiliary Manifestations

Between 2 and 4% of patients with UC and a smaller proportion of those with CD have associated PSC. It should be noted that 50–80% or more of patients may exhibit mildly elevated alkaline phosphatase, reflecting pericholangitis presumed to be at the very mildest end of the continuum of PSC. In contrast, nearly 80% of patients with PSC have underlying IBD, mostly UC. Consequently, a diagnostic colonoscopy is recommended in patients diagnosed with PSC even in the absence of underlying bowel symptoms, as asymptomatic colitis is seen in a significant fraction and has implications for colorectal cancer risk. Smoking appears to be protective against PSC independent of its inverse association with UC. Recent genome-wide association studies (GWAS) identified several loci associated with PSC, including human leukocyte antigen (HLA) on chromosome 6p21 and rs9524260 at chromosome 13q31 [20]. Two of the UC loci (2q35 and 3p21) were also found associated with PSC, suggesting shared genetic risk [20].

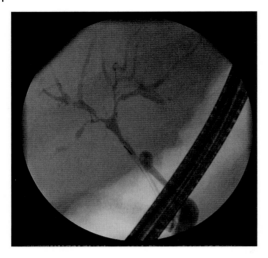

**Figure 4.4** Endoscopic retrograde cholangiographic image of a patient with PSC demonstrating beading and dilation of the intrahepatic ducts.

Serum alkaline phosphatase is elevated in most patients with PSC and persistently elevated alkaline phosphatase levels should trigger further evaluation for PSC. The diagnosis is usually made by magnetic resonance cholangiopancreatography (MRCP). An endoscopic retrograde cholangiopancreatography (ERCP) exam is now reserved mainly for therapeutic interventions such as those with a dominant stricture or with suspicion of cholangiocarcinoma (Figure 4.4). Rarely, a liver biopsy may be needed to establish diagnosis, particularly in patients with small duct PSC where there may be no large duct changes visible on imaging. The classic liver histology described in PSC is periductal inflammation, fibrosis, and obliteration of the bile ducts, resulting in an "onion-skin" appearance. Progressive PSC can lead to biliary strictures and cholangitis. Dominant biliary strictures can be managed with balloon dilation or stent placement. PSC can lead to progressive fibrosis, cirrhosis, and portal hypertension, ultimately requiring liver transplantation.

The underlying bowel disease in IBD–PSC demonstrates a greater proportion of pancolitis in both UC and CD, less frequent ileal involvement, and a milder natural history [21]. Recent studies suggested that a milder course of PSC may be associated with higher rates of colectomy and more severe bowel disease whereas more aggressive PSC leading to liver transplantation may be associated with milder bowel disease [22]. Among patients undergoing colectomy with an ileal pouch anal anastomosis (IPAA), there is an increased risk of pouchitis [22]. The occurrence of IBD and PSC may not be concurrent in all patients as the bowel disease can develop only after liver transplantation for PSC, while conversely, PSC can manifest itself after colectomy in IBD [22]. Patients with PSC have a significantly greater risk of colorectal cancer compared with those without [23, 24] and should be entered into an annual colonoscopic surveillance program. As this risk persists even after liver transplantation, surveillance should continue in such patients [25]. The role of ursodeoxycholic acid (UDCA) in the management of PSC is controversial. An initial case–control study suggested a chemoprotective effect with a dose of 13–15 mg kg$^{-1}$ per day [26]. However, a study utilizing a higher dose of UDCA (28–30 mg kg$^{-1}$ per day) suggested increased risk of liver disease progression and colorectal neoplasia [27].

Patients with IBD can also experience other hepatobiliary diseases, including hepatic steatosis, steatohepatitis, and cholelithiasis. Drug-induced liver injury may occur in patients with IBD associated with the use of thiopurines, methotrexate, or antibiotics. Rarely, liver injury has also been reported with anti-TNF use [28]. Patients with ileal Crohn's disease are at risk for both cholesterol and pigment gallstones. Bile acid malabsorption and depletion leads to reduced hepatic secretion of bile acids and supersaturation of bile, resulting in cholesterol gallstones. In addition, bile acid malabsorption leading to solubilization of unconjugated bilirubin in the colon may result in greater reabsorption and transport to the liver, leading to precipitation and formation of pigment gallstones [29].

## Ophthalmologic Manifestations

Ocular manifestations occur in up to 10% of patients with IBD and present as episcleritis, scleritis, uveitis, or iritis. Rarer manifestations include optic neuropathy, vaso-occlusive phenomena, posterior choroiditis, vasculitis, and intraretinal hemorrhage [30]. Additional ocular findings include those related to treatment complications such as glaucoma and cataracts from corticosteroid use. Similarly to the other EIMs, ocular manifestations can occur in conjunction with bowel disease or joint symptoms. The main clinical presentation is redness of the eye, blurred vision, pain, photophobia, or headaches. Diagnosis is made clinically and by ophthalmologic examination under a slit-lamp. Permanent visual damage due to repeated inflammatory episodes may occur but is uncommon. Some ocular manifestations such as episcleritis parallel bowel disease and respond to treatment of the underlying bowel symptoms or topical corticosteroids. In contrast, scleritis, a more severe disease, is independent of activity of bowel symptoms. Uveitis presents as redness and photophobia and may occur in association with bowel and joint symptoms, although it is frequently independent of both and may even precede the diagnosis of IBD (Figure 4.5). Treatment involves topical steroids, cycloplegics, and occasionally systemic steroids. Case series suggest good efficacy with the use of anti-TNF therapy and systemic immunosuppression [31, 32].

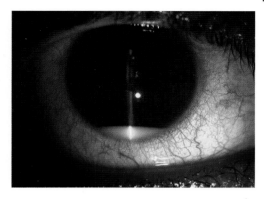

**Figure 4.5** Uveitis in a patient with inflammatory bowel disease.

## Renal Complications

The primary renal complication associated with IBD is nephrolithiasis. Between 12 and 28% of patients with IBD have nephrolithiasis compared with 5% of the general population. This risk is higher in patients with CD, particularly in those with ileocolonic disease [33]. The renal stones in patients with CD are most commonly calcium oxalate stones. The bile salt and fat malabsorption that occurs due to ileal disease or following ileal resection leads to increased binding of calcium to the free fatty acids, resulting in higher free oxalate levels in the gut as oxalate is normally complexed with the calcium. This oxalate is absorbed in the colon and leads to increased serum oxalate levels, hyperoxaluria, and consequently oxalate stones. Prevention of oxalate stones can be facilitated by oral calcium supplementation and a low-oxalate diet. The second most common type of stone in IBD is uric acid stones. These usually develop in people with volume depletion, particularly with an ileostomy. Uric acid stones can be prevented by alkalinization of the urine with the use of potassium citrate.

Chronic inflammation may lead to amyloidosis, which can present as proteinuria and renal insufficiency. Treatment of underlying IBD can rarely stop disease progression by controlling the inflammation. Some of the medications used in the management of IBD can also lead to renal toxicity. Interstitial nephritis is a well-recognized but rare side effect of 5-aminosalicylate use. Serum creatinine should be measured every 12 months in patients on these medications and annual urinalysis will assess proteinuria. Dose-dependent nephrotoxicity is a well recognized complication of cyclosporine and tacrolimus use. Other medications such as thiopurines may need a dose reduction in the setting of significant renal failure.

## Thromboembolic and Cardiovascular Complications

IBD is a well-recognized risk factor for venous thromboembolism (VTE) [34–36]. In a large cohort study, IBD was associated with a twofold increase in risk of all VTE and unprovoked VTE. This relative risk was greater in younger patients and those who were ambulatory whereas the absolute risk of VTE was highest among the hospitalized [34]. Consequently, all hospitalized patients with IBD should receive routine thromboprophylaxis unless a strong contraindication exists. Prophylactic anticoagulation appears to be well tolerated even in the setting of ongoing mild to moderate gastrointestinal blood loss due to IBD. Inherited thrombophilias are not more common in patients with IBD and do not contribute to this excess risk. However, ongoing inflammation appears to be an important driver of VTE risk [36], with both hospitalized and ambulatory flares being associated with an increased risk [36, 37]. Most of the VTE events are deep venous thrombosis or pulmonary embolism. However, thrombosis at unusual sites, such as mesenteric vein thrombosis or portal vein thrombosis, can occur. Thromboprophylaxis is safe even in patients hospitalized with overt bleeding. The management of VTE events in patients with IBD is similar to that in the general populations. However, given the prothrombotic nature of IBD, the optimal duration of anticoagulation has not been adequately defined. Routine extended anticoagulation beyond discharge [38] or primary prophylaxis during ambulatory flares does not appear to be cost-effective [39].

The effect of IBD on arterial thromboembolic risk is less certain. Elevated cardiovascular disease risk has been demonstrated in some subgroups of patients with IBD. A recent meta-analysis identified a modest increase in risk of cerebrovascular accidents and ischemic heart disease in IBD, but primarily among women, and in younger patients.

## Case Studies and Multiple Choice Questions

1  Michael is a 25-year-old man with ulcerative pancolitis who is being treated with mesalamine 4.8 g per day. For the past 5 months, he has been noticing lower back pain that is associated with stiffness in the mornings and improvement during the course of the day. He runs 3 miles daily and has not noted any worsening of the pain with exercise. His primary care provider obtained a plain X ray of the lumbar spine which revealed sacroileitis. Which of the following statements is true about this condition?

   A  Low back pain related to sacroileitis strongly correlates with ongoing activity of luminal colonic IBD.
   B  The course of sacroileitis is frequently independent of the presence of inflammatory activity in the colon.
   C  Nearly all patients with IBD who develop sacroileitis will progress to ankylosing spondylitis.
   D  NOD2 positivity is more common in those with sacroiliac inflammation in IBD.

2  Which of the following treatments are not effective in the management of peristomal pyoderma gangrenosum in patients with IBD?

   A  Topical corticosteroids.
   B  Oral cyclopsorine.
   C  Anti-TNF biologic therapy.
   D  Oral mesalamine.

3  Which is the appropriate colorectal neoplasia surveillance interval for patients with IBD and coexisting primary sclerosing cholangitis?

   A  Annual surveillance colonoscopy from diagnosis.
   B  Fecal occult blood test annually and colonoscopy every 2 years.
   C  Colonoscopy every 5 years.
   D  Colonoscopy annually beginning 8 years after diagnosis.

4  Mark is a 63-year-old man with a history of refractory ulcerative colitis for which he underwent a total proctocolectomy with an end-ileostomy 10 years ago. Which of the following types of renal stones are more common in Mark?

   A  Calcium oxalate.
   B  Uric acid.
   C  Struvite.
   D  Cystine.

# References

1 Atzeni, F., Defendenti, C., Ditto, M.C., *et al.* (2014) Rheumatic manifestations in inflammatory bowel disease. *Autoimmunity Reviews*, **13**(1), 20–23.

2 Orchard, T.R., Wordsworth, B.P., and Jewell, D.P. (1998) Peripheral arthropathies in inflammatory bowel disease: their articular distribution and natural history. *Gut*, **42**(3), 387–391.

3 Orchard, T.R., Thiyagaraja, S., Welsh, K.I., *et al.* (2000) Clinical phenotype is related to HLA genotype in the peripheral arthropathies of inflammatory bowel disease. *Gastroenterology*, **118**(2), 274–278.

4 Rudwaleit, M. and Baeten, D. (2006) Ankylosing spondylitis and bowel disease. *Best Practice & Research. Clinical Rheumatology*, **20**(3), 451–471.

5 McLeod, C., Bagust, A., Boland, A., *et al.* (2007) Adalimumab, etanercept and infliximab for the treatment of ankylosing spondylitis: a systematic review and economic evaluation. *Health Technology Assessment*, **11**(28), 1–158, iii–iv.

6 Targownik, L.E., Bernstein, C.N., Nugent, Z., and Leslie, W.D. (2013) Inflammatory bowel disease has a small effect on bone mineral density and risk for osteoporosis. *Clinical Gastroenterology and Hepatology*, **11**(3), 278–285.

7 Vazquez, M.A., Lopez, E., Montoya, M.J., *et al.* (2012) Vertebral fractures in patients with inflammatory bowel disease compared with a healthy population: a prospective case–control study. *BMC Gastroenterology*, **12**, 47.

8 Weiss, R.J., Wick, M.C., Ackermann, P.W., and Montgomery, S.M. (2010) Increased fracture risk in patients with rheumatic disorders and other inflammatory diseases – a case–control study with 53,108 patients with fracture. *Journal of Rheumatology*, **37**(11), 2247–2250.

9 Vestergaard, P., Krogh, K., Rejnmark, L., *et al.* (2000) Fracture risk is increased in Crohn's disease, but not in ulcerative colitis. *Gut*, **46**(2), 176–181.

10 Targownik, L.E., Bernstein, C.N., Nugent, Z., *et al.* (2013) Inflammatory bowel disease and the risk of fracture after controlling for FRAX. *Journal of Bone and Mineral Research*, **28**(5), 1007–1013.

11 Kappelman, M.D., Galanko, J.A., Porter, C.Q., and Sandler, R.S. (2011) Risk of diagnosed fractures in children with inflammatory bowel diseases. *Inflammatory Bowel Diseases*, **17**(5), 1125–1130.

12 Loftus, E.V., Jr., Crowson, C.S., Sandborn, W.J., *et al.* (2002) Long-term fracture risk in patients with Crohn's disease: a population-based study in Olmsted County, Minnesota. *Gastroenterology*, **123**(2), 468–475.

13 Loftus, E.V., Jr., Achenbach, S.J., Sandborn, W.J., *et al.* (2003) Risk of fracture in ulcerative colitis: a population-based study from Olmsted County, Minnesota. *Clinical Gastroenterology and Hepatology*, **1**(6), 465–473.

14 American Gastroenterological Association (2003) American Gastroenterological Association medical

position statement: guidelines on osteoporosis in gastrointestinal diseases. *Gastroenterology*, **124**(3), 791–794.

15  Melek, J. and Sakuraba, A. (2014) Efficacy and safety of medical therapy for low bone-mineral density in patients with inflammatory bowel disease: a meta-analysis and systematic review. *Clinical Gastroenterology and Hepatology*, **12**(1), 32–44.e5.

16  Agarwal, A. and Andrews, J.M. (2013) Systematic review: IBD-associated pyoderma gangrenosum in the biologic era, the response to therapy. *Alimentary Pharmacology & Therapeutics*, **38**(6), 563–572.

17  Cullen, G., Kroshinsky, D., Cheifetz, A.S., and Korzenik, J.R. (2011) Psoriasis associated with anti-tumour necrosis factor therapy in inflammatory bowel disease: a new series and a review of 120 cases from the literature. *Alimentary Pharmacology & Therapeutics*, **34**(11–12), 1318–1327.

18  Rahier, J.F., Buche, S., Peyrin-Biroulet, L., *et al.* (2010) Severe skin lesions cause patients with inflammatory bowel disease to discontinue anti-tumor necrosis factor therapy. *Clinical Gastroenterology and Hepatology*, **8**(12), 1048–1055.

19  de Gannes, G.C., Ghoreishi, M., Pope, J., *et al.* (2007) Psoriasis and pustular dermatitis triggered by TNF-α inhibitors in patients with rheumatologic conditions. *Archives of Dermatology*, **143**(2), 223–231.

20  Karlsen, T.H., Franke, A., Melum, E., *et al.* (2010) Genome-wide association analysis in primary sclerosing cholangitis. *Gastroenterology*, **138**(3), 1102–1111.

21  Loftus, E.V., Jr., Harewood, G.C., Loftus, C.G., *et al.* (2005) PSC–IBD: a unique form of inflammatory bowel disease associated with primary sclerosing cholangitis. *Gut*, **54**(1), 91–96.

22  Eaton, J.E., Talwalkar, J.A., Lazaridis, K.N., *et al.* (2013) Pathogenesis of primary sclerosing cholangitis and advances in diagnosis and management. *Gastroenterology*, **145**(3), 521–536.

23  Loftus, E.V., Jr. (2006) Epidemiology and risk factors for colorectal dysplasia and cancer in ulcerative colitis. *Gastroenterology Clinics of North America*, **35**(3), 517–531.

24  Jess, T., Loftus, E.V., Jr., Velayos, F.S., *et al.* (2007) Risk factors for colorectal neoplasia in inflammatory bowel disease: a nested case–control study from Copenhagen county, Denmark and Olmsted county, Minnesota. *American Journal of Gastroenterology*, **102**(4), 829–836.

25  Singh, S., Varayil, J.E., Loftus, E.V., Jr., and Talwalkar, J.A. (2013) Incidence of colorectal cancer after liver transplantation for primary sclerosing cholangitis: a systematic review and meta-analysis. *Liver Transplantation*, **19**(12), 1361–1369.

26  Pardi, D.S., Loftus, E.V., Jr., Kremers, W.K., *et al.* (2003) Ursodeoxycholic acid as a chemopreventive agent in patients with ulcerative colitis and primary sclerosing cholangitis. *Gastroenterology*, **124**(4), 889–893.

27  Eaton, J.E., Silveira, M.G., Pardi, D.S., *et al.* (2011) High-dose ursodeoxycholic acid is associated with the development of colorectal neoplasia in patients with ulcerative colitis and primary sclerosing cholangitis. *American Journal of Gastroenterology*, **106**(9), 1638–1645.

28  Sokolove, J., Strand, V., Greenberg, J.D., *et al.* (2010) Risk of elevated liver enzymes associated with TNF inhibitor utilisation in patients with rheumatoid arthritis. *Annals of the Rheumatic Diseases*, **69**(9), 1612–1617.

29  Stinton, L.M. and Shaffer, E.A. (2012) Epidemiology of gallbladder disease: cholelithiasis and cancer. *Gut Liver*, **6**(2), 172–187.

30  Calvo, P. and Pablo, L. (2013) Managing IBD outside the gut: ocular manifestations. *Digestive Diseases*, **31**(2), 229–232.

31  Kruh, J.N., Yang, P., Suelves, A.M., and Foster, C.S. (2014) Infliximab for the treatment of refractory noninfectious uveitis: a study of 88 patients with

long-term follow-up. *Ophthalmology*, **121**(1), 358–364.

32 Murphy, C.C., Ayliffe, W.H., Booth, A., *et al.* (2004) Tumor necrosis factor alpha blockade with infliximab for refractory uveitis and scleritis. *Ophthalmology*, **111**(2), 352–356.

33 Oikonomou, K., Kapsoritakis, A., Eleftheriadis, T., *et al.* (2011) Renal manifestations and complications of inflammatory bowel disease. *Inflammatory Bowel Diseases*, **17**(4), 1034–1045.

34 Kappelman, M.D., Horvath-Puho, E., Sandler, R.S., *et al.* (2011) Thromboembolic risk among Danish children and adults with inflammatory bowel diseases: a population-based nationwide study. *Gut*, **60**(7), 937–943.

35 Bernstein, C.N., Blanchard, J.F., Houston, D.S., and Wajda, A. (2001) The incidence of deep venous thrombosis and pulmonary embolism among patients with inflammatory bowel disease: a population-based cohort study. *Thrombosis and Haemostasis*, **85**(3), 430–434.

36 Grainge, M.J., West, J., and Card, T.R. (2010) Venous thromboembolism during active disease and remission in inflammatory bowel disease: a cohort study. *Lancet*, **375**(9715), 657–663.

37 Murthy, S.K. and Nguyen, G.C. (2011) Venous thromboembolism in inflammatory bowel disease: an epidemiological review. *American Journal of Gastroenterology*, **106**(4), 713–718.

38 Nguyen, G.C. and Bernstein, C.N. (2013) Duration of anticoagulation for the management of venous thromboembolism in inflammatory bowel disease: a decision analysis. *American Journal of Gastroenterology*, **108**(9), 1486–1495.

39 Nguyen, G.C. and Sharma, S. (2013) Feasibility of venous thromboembolism prophylaxis during inflammatory bowel disease flares in the outpatient setting: a decision analysis. *Inflammatory Bowel Diseases*, **19**(10), 2182–2189.

## Answers to Questions

1 Answer: **B**. Sacroileitis is seen in 2–32% of patients with IBD and presents typically as low back pain with morning stiffness that is relieved by physical activity. It is frequently but not always independent of underlying bowel disease activity [4]. In contrast, type 1 peripheral arthropathy involving the large joints such as the elbows and knees frequently parallels inflammatory activity in the intestine.

2 Answer: **D**. Pyoderma gangrenosum occurs in 1–5% of patients with IBD and typically presents as an ulcer with a necrotic base and progressive destruction. The first-line treatment is topical or intralesional corticosteroids and wound care. In those with refractory disease, systemic treatment with anti-TNF agents, corticosteroids, or cyclosporine may be required. Mesalamine derivatives have not been demonstrated to be effective in the management of peristomal pyoderma.

3 Answer: **A**. Patients with PSC and UC have an increased risk of colorectal cancer compared with those without PSC [23, 24] and should be entered into an annual colonoscopic surveillance program from the time of diagnosis. As the risk persists, surveillance should continue even after liver transplantation [25].

4 Answer: **B**. Patients with an ileostomy are more prone to volume depletion, which is associated with uric acid stones. This can be prevented by alkalinization of urine with potassium citrate. In contrast, those with ileal Crohn's disease are more likely to have calcium oxalate stones due to bile salt and fat malabsorption (provided that the colon is intact, as the latter is the site of calcium oxalate absorption).

# Section II

# Therapeutic Agents

# 5

# Aminosalicylates

## Clinical Take Home Messages

- Several 5-aminosalicylate (5-ASA) preparations, both oral and topical, are available for the treatment of inflammatory bowel diseases. The moiety to which it is conjugated influences properties related to delivery of 5-ASA as the active agent, in addition to usual dose and frequency of administration.
- Aminosalicylates in doses of 2.4–4.8 g per day of mesalamine or equivalent are efficacious in inducing remission in mild to moderate ulcerative colitis.
- There may be a dose response, with greater efficacy of the 4.8 g per day dose in those with moderate severity of ulcerative colitis, whereas all doses above 2 g per day may be equally effective in mild disease.
- Data suggest that aminosalicylates have limited effectiveness in inducing or maintaining remission in Crohn's disease.

Aminosalicylates were the first medications demonstrated to have efficacy for ulcerative colitis (UC). Sulfasalazine, the first drug in this class developed, is a combination of sulfapyridine, an antibiotic, and 5-aminosalicylic acid (5-ASA), an anti-inflammatory agent. However, it was soon recognized that the active moiety was not sulfapyridine but the 5-ASA component. Subsequently, several different formulations of 5-ASA were developed, with varying mechanisms of drug delivery and site of release within the gastrointestinal tract. A majority of the effects of 5-ASA drugs are from their topical action in the colon, as less than one-third is absorbed into the systemic circulation. For example, after ingestion, sulfasalazine undergoes metabolism in the colon by the bacterial azoreductase enzymes into 5-ASA and sulfapyridine. Several different mechanisms of action have been proposed to explain the efficacy of these agents. Thus, they may block interleukin-1 and tumor necrosis factor alpha (TNF-α) by inhibiting the binding of TNF-α to its receptor, preventing downstream signaling [1–4]. In addition, 5-ASA may activate the peroxisome proliferator-activated receptors (PPARs) in the colonic epithelium, and inhibit production of prostaglandin $E_2$ through the arachidonic acid pathway. It may also act as a free radical scavenger [4].

Both oral and topical aminosalicylate formulations are available. Owing to poor systemic absorption, the efficacy of oral formulations depends on achieving an adequate luminal concentration of 5-ASA at the site of active disease. Oral agents are effective for both pancolitis and limited distal colitis and topical agents administered per rectum are used only for distal disease. Several different 5-ASA formulations are available in the United States and Europe. They vary in recommended doses and strength of individual capsules. In addition, the delivery mechanism and site of release of the active 5-ASA moiety vary among the preparations (Table 5.1). As noted above, sulfasalazine consists of a 5-ASA moiety linked to sulfapyridine by an azo bond cleaved by colonic bacterial azoreductase and thus is only suitable for colonic disease. Asacol consists of 5-ASA enclosed in an enteric coated film (Eudragit-S) and is released at pH ≥7 in the distal ileum and colon. A derivative of this, Lialda, incorporates a multi-matrix release system allowing for once per day administration of the drug. Olsalazine consists of two molecules of 5-ASA linked by an azo bond and is released in the distal small bowel and colon.

Balsalazide is comprised of 5-ASA linked to an inactive carrier and is released in the right colon. In contrast, Pentasa uses ethylcellulose-coated granules that release 5-ASA at pH ≥6, delivering approximately half of the 5-ASA in the small intestine, and is an option for the treatment of small bowel inflammation.

## Efficacy in Ulcerative Colitis

Most trials of aminosalicylates have been conducted in patients with mild to moderate UC and have demonstrated efficacy in both induction and maintenance of remission. The efficacy of sulfasalazine in the management of UC was first reported in 1942 by Svartz [5]. Subsequent randomized controlled trials (RCTs) demonstrated efficacy of sulfasalazine in the induction of remission in mild to moderate UC. Topical sulfasalazine treatment (3 g per day sulfasalazine enema) was also effective in patients with

Table 5.1 Preparations of 5-aminosalicylic acid derivatives in the United States.

| Product | Formulation | Size of tablets (mg) | Typical dose | Site of release |
|---|---|---|---|---|
| Sulfasalazine | 5-ASA linked to sulfapyridine | 500 | 2–6 g per day; t.i.d.–q.i.d. | Colon |
| Asacol, Delzicol | 5-ASA coated with Eudragit-S resin; release at pH ≥7 | 400 | 2.4–4.8 g per day; q.d.–b.i.d. | Distal ileum; colon |
| Asacol HD | 5-ASA coated with Eudragit-S resin; release at pH ≥7 | 800 | 2.4–4.8 g per day; q.d.–b.i.d. | Distal ileum; colon |
| Lialda | 5-ASA coated with multi-matrix and Eudragit-S resin; release at pH ≥7 | 1200 | 2.4–4.8 g per day; q.d.–b.i.d. | Distal ileum; colon |
| Apriso | 5-ASA coated with Eudragit-L coating released at pH ≥6, and polymer matrix core facilitating slow release throughout the colon | 375 | 1.5 g per day; q.d. | Ileum and colon |
| Pentasa | Microspheres with a moisture-sensitive ethylcellulose coating | 250, 500 | 3–4 g per day; b.i.d.–q.i.d. | Duodenum, jejunum, ileum, colon |
| Olsalazine | 5-ASA dimer linked by an azo bond | 250 | 1–2 g per day; b.i.d. | Colon |
| Balsalazide | 5-ASA linked to an inert carrier | 750 | 6.75 g per day; b.i.d.–t.i.d. | Colon |

ulcerative proctitis. Oral sulfasalazine is usually dosed at 1–4 g per day, not exceeding a daily dose of 6 g. Oral corticosteroids are more effective and act faster than sulfasalazine.

Mesalamine is effective in both induction and maintenance of remission in UC [6]. A meta-analysis of 11 RCTs demonstrated remission in 60% of patients after 8 weeks of treatment compared with 20% receiving placebo. Specifically restricting the analysis to 1722 patients on mesalamine, there was a lower rate of failure to achieve remission with mesalamine treatment compared with placebo [relative risk (RR) 0.79, 95% confidence interval (CI) 0.71–0.88] and its efficacy was similar to that of sulfasalazine and other aminosalicylates, suggesting that as a drug class, the efficacy of each individual agent is similar at comparable doses and there may be limited benefit of switching drugs within the same class in the setting of lack of efficacy [7]. The standard dose of mesalamine for induction of remission is 2.4–4.8 g per day. For milder disease, both doses appear to have comparable efficacy, whereas for moderate disease, the higher dose produces greater benefit. In the ASCEND I trial including 301 patients with mild to moderate UC randomized to 2.4 or 4.8 g per day, at 6 weeks the overall

improvement, defined as clinical remission or response, was no different between the two groups (51% vs. 56%). However, in those with moderate disease, 72% of patients responded with the 4.8 g per day dose compared with 57% with the 2.4 g per day dose (Figure 5.1) [8]. This was confirmed in a second RCT [9]. Once per day dosing is similar to conventional dosing in terms of efficacy; as an alternative it may yield better patient compliance [10]. Other oral 5-ASA agents have also been studied in UC. Olsalazine at doses of 1–2 g per day and balsalazide at 6.75 g per day have efficacy similar to that of mesalamine or sulfasalazine.

Topical (per rectum) formulations of 5-ASA include suppositories, foams, and enemas. Mesalamine suppositories are usually administered in doses of 1 g per day whereas enemas are formulated as 4 g per day preparations. Rectal suppositories deliver adequate luminal concentrations of 5-ASA to the distal 15–20 cm of the rectum, whereas enemas may reach the level of the splenic flexure. In patients with limited distal colitis, rectal 5-ASA preparations are more efficacious than topical corticosteroid therapy. Rectal 5-ASA may also have greater efficacy than oral 5-ASA therapy in patients with

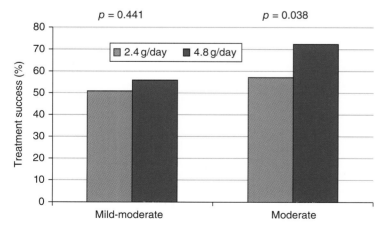

**Figure 5.1** Dose response to delayed release oral mesalamine (4.8 g per day compared with 2.4 g per day) in mild to -moderate ulcerative colitis. *Source:* Adapted from Hanauer *et al.* 2007 [8].

isolated proctitis or proctosigmoiditis and yield faster resolution of symptoms [11, 12].

Aminosalicylates are not effective in the treatment of severe colitis. Owing to the risk of paradoxical worsening of colitis, the use of aminosalicylates is usually interrupted in patients with severe disease, particularly with recent initiation of 5-ASA therapy. Rectal 5-ASA preparations may be less well tolerated that topical corticosteroids with severe disease.

## Efficacy in Crohn's Disease

There are far fewer data supporting the efficacy of aminosalicylates in Crohn's disease (CD). In the National Cooperative Crohn's Disease Study (NCCDS), which randomized patients to sulfasalazine, azathioprine, or prednisone, those randomized to sulfasalazine had superior response compared with placebo at 4 months [13]. However, this benefit was restricted to patients with colonic or ileocolonic disease; no efficacy was found in patients with isolated ileal disease. These findings were confirmed by the European Cooperative Crohn's Disease Study (ECCDS), in which sulfasalazine was superior to placebo for colonic CD, but inferior to prednisone in all patient groups [14]. The restriction of effect to colonic CD may be attributable to the requirement for colonic bacterial azoreductase to release the 5-ASA moiety. Seven placebo-controlled trials examined the efficacy of mesalamine formulations in the treatment of mild to moderate CD. A meta-analysis of 647 patients enrolled in the eligible treatment trials demonstrated no difference in the likelihood of induction remission with mesalamine compared with placebo in active CD. Multiple trials have examined the efficacy of mesalamine for maintenance of corticosteroid-induced remission in CD, but most failed to find a benefit to their use, or found

only modest effects on the maintenance of remission. Two trials of sulfasalazine for preventing relapse in quiescent CD found no benefit with therapy (RR 0.98, 95% CI 0.82–1.17) [15]. In contrast, among the 11 trials encompassing 1753 patients randomized to mesalamine or placebo, the rate of relapse was modestly lower among the mesalamine group (53% vs. 57%; RR 0.94, 95% CI 0.87–1.01).

## Safety

Side effects are common with sulfasalazine, occurring in about one-third of patients at a dose of 4 g per day. Side effects of sulfasalazine (as opposed to other aminosalicylates) may be dose related. Common adverse effects include nausea, vomiting, abdominal pain, headaches, skin rash, fever, liver enzyme abnormalities, and, less commonly, aplastic anemia, leucopenia, or agranulocytosis. Folic acid deficiency is a well-recognized consequence of sulfasalazine use and patients on long-term sulfasalazine maintenance should be supplemented with 1 mg per day of folic acid. Sulfasalazine can also cause low sperm counts in men; patients on sulfasalazine may switch to an alternative 5-ASA if planning conception. Owing to the highly absorbed sulfapyridine moiety, sulfasalazine should be avoided in patients with known hypersensitivity to sulfa drugs.

Two adverse reactions are specific to the aminosalicylates. A small minority (<5%) of patients initiating therapy may experience a paradoxical worsening of their symptoms characterized by abdominal pain, diarrhea, rectal bleeding, and fever. This can be seen with any 5-ASA preparation, oral or topical, and recurs with any other drug in this category. Interstitial nephritis, the second rare side effect, is observed in fewer than 0.3% of patients. A prospective study using data from the United Kingdom General Practice

Research Database following 19 025 5-ASA users identified no increase in risk of renal disease in current users of 5-ASA [odds ratio (OR) 0.86, 95% CI 0.53–1.41] and a modest increase in risk in recent users (OR 2.48, 95% CI 1.33–4.61) [16]. Only a few cases of interstitial nephritis were associated with 5-ASA use. However, most practitioners advocate monitoring renal function by annual urinalysis screen for proteinuria in patients with ongoing 5-ASA therapy. Most cases of 5-ASA-induced interstitial nephritis resolve with drug withdrawal and rarely require steroid use [17]. Other rare adverse effects of 5-ASA therapy include pericarditis, myocarditis, pneumonitis, pancreatitis, and hepatitis. Azo-containing 5-ASA derivatives have been associated with diarrhea in 5–10% of patients due to induction of chloride secretion in the small intestine.

## Multiple Choice Questions

1  Which of the following side effects have not been reported with aminosalicylates?
   A  Increased risk of *Clostridium difficile* infection.
   B  Interstitial nephritis.
   C  Pancreatitis.
   D  Paradoxical worsening of colitis.

2  Which of the following statements is true about paradoxical worsening of colitis with aminosalicylate therapy?
   A  It is a drug-specific effect and will not recur with use of a different aminosalicylate agent.
   B  It is seen only with oral therapy and does not occur with use of topical aminosalicylates.

   C  It occurs only in patients with severe colitis and is not seen in those with milder disease.
   D  It is seen only with sulfasalazine in patients who are allergic to sulfa medications.
   E  None of the above.

3  Which of the following micronutrient supplements those using sulfasalazine therapy should routinely take?
   A  Calcium and vitamin D.
   B  Vitamin $B_{12}$.
   C  Folic acid.
   D  Magnesium.

# References

1 Rachmilewitz, D., Karmeli, F., Schwartz, L.W., and Simon, P.L. (1992) Effect of aminophenols (5-ASA and 4-ASA) on colonic interleukin-1 generation. *Gut*, **33**(7), 929–932.

2 Mahida, Y.R., Lamming, C.E., Gallagher, A., *et al.* (1991) 5-Aminosalicylic acid is a potent inhibitor of interleukin 1 beta production in organ culture of colonic biopsy specimens from patients with inflammatory bowel disease. *Gut*, **32**(1), 50–54.

3 Desreumaux, P. and Ghosh, S. (2006) Review article: mode of action and delivery of 5-aminosalicylic acid – new evidence. *Alimentary Pharmacology & Therapeutics*, **24**(Suppl. 1), 2–9.

4 Sonu, I., Lin, M.V., Blonski, W., and Lichtenstein, G.R. (2010) Clinical pharmacology of 5-ASA compounds in inflammatory bowel disease. *Gastroenterology Clinics of North America*, **39**(3), 559–599.

5 Svartz, N. (1988) Sulfasalazine: II. Some notes on the discovery and development of salazopyrin. *American Journal of Gastroenterology*, **83**(5), 497–503.

6 Ford, A.C., Achkar, J.P., Khan, K.J., *et al.* (2011) Efficacy of 5-aminosalicylates in ulcerative colitis: systematic review and meta-analysis. *American Journal of Gastroenterology*, **106**(4), 601–616.

7 Feagan, B.G. and Macdonald, J.K. (2012) Oral 5-aminosalicylic acid for induction of remission in ulcerative colitis. *Cochrane Database of Systematic Reviews*, (**10**), CD000543.

8 Hanauer, S.B., Sandborn, W.J., Dallaire, C., *et al.* (2007) Delayed-release oral mesalamine 4.8 g/day (800 mg tablets) compared to 2.4 g/day (400 mg tablets) for the treatment of mildly to moderately active ulcerative colitis: The ASCEND I trial. *Canadian Journal of Gastroenterology = Journal Canadien de Gastroenterologie*, **21**(12), 827–834.

9 Hanauer, S.B., Sandborn, W.J., Kornbluth, A., *et al.* (2005) Delayed-release oral mesalamine at 4.8 g/day (800 mg tablet) for the treatment of moderately active ulcerative colitis: the ASCEND II trial. *American Journal of Gastroenterology*, **100**(11), 2478–2485.

10 Ford, A.C., Khan, K.J., Sandborn, W.J., *et al.* (2011) Once-daily dosing vs. conventional dosing schedule of mesalamine and relapse of quiescent ulcerative colitis: systematic review and meta-analysis. *American Journal of Gastroenterology*, **106**(12), 2070–2077; quiz, 2078.

11 Safdi, M., DeMicco, M., Sninsky, C., *et al.* (1997) A double-blind comparison of oral versus rectal mesalamine versus combination therapy in the treatment of distal ulcerative colitis. *American Journal of Gastroenterology*, **92**(10), 1867–1871.

12 Ford, A.C., Khan, K.J., Achkar, J.P., and Moayyedi, P. (2012) Efficacy of oral vs. topical, or combined oral and topical 5-aminosalicylates, in ulcerative colitis: systematic review and meta-analysis.

*American Journal of Gastroenterology*, **107**(2), 167–176; author reply, 177.

13 Summers, R.W., Switz, D.M., Sessions, J.T., Jr., *et al.* (1979) National Cooperative Crohn's Disease Study: results of drug treatment. *Gastroenterology*, **77**(4 Pt. 2), 847–869.

14 Malchow, H., Ewe, K., Brandes, J.W., *et al.* (1984) European Cooperative Crohn's Disease Study (ECCDS): results of drug treatment. *Gastroenterology*, **86**(2), 249–266.

15 Ford, A.C., Kane, S.V., Khan, K.J., *et al.* (2011) Efficacy of 5-aminosalicylates in Crohn's disease: systematic review and meta-analysis. *American Journal of Gastroenterology*, **106**(4), 617–629.

16 Van Staa, T.P., Travis, S., Leufkens, H.G.M., and Logan, R.F. (2004) 5-Aminosalicylic acids and the risk of renal disease: a large British epidemiologic study. *Gastroenterology*, **126**(7), 1733–1739.

17 Gisbert, J.P., Gonzalez-Lama, Y., and Mate, J. (2007) 5-Aminosalicylates and renal function in inflammatory bowel disease: a systematic review. *Inflammatory Bowel Diseases*, **13**(5), 629–638.

## Answers to Questions

1   Answer: A. Owing to their non-immuno-suppressive mechanism of action, amino-salicylates have not been associated with an increased risk of infections or immu-nosuppression-related malignancies.

2   Answer: E. Paradoxical worsening of colitis is a class effect and can be seen with any aminosalicylate therapy. Thus its occurrence represents a contraindi-cation to future use of any oral or topi-cal aminosalicylate. The likelihood of paradoxical worsening is independent of the severity of underlying IBD and it does not represent an allergic reaction to the sulfa moiety, in contrast to other hyper-sensitivity reactions to sulfasalazine.

3   Answer: C. Folic acid deficiency is a well-recognized consequence of sulfasalazine use and patients on long-term sulfasalazine maintenance should be supplemented with 1 mg per day of folic acid.

# 6

# Corticosteroids

---

## Clinical Take Home Messages

- Systemic corticosteroids are efficacious in the induction of remission in patients with moderate to severe ulcerative colitis (UC), acute severe fulminant colitis, and moderate to severe Crohn's disease (CD).
- Non-systemic corticosteroids (budesonide) are also effective in inducing remission in both CD and UC, are inferior in efficacy to systemic corticosteroids, but may have fewer systemic adverse effects
- Long-term use of corticosteroids is not recommended for maintenance of remission in CD or UC owing to a range of reversible and irreversible adverse effects. Up to two-thirds of patients either become dependent on steroids or develop refractory disease.

---

Systemic corticosteroids are efficacious in the induction of remission in patients with moderate to severe ulcerative colitis (UC), acute severe fulminant colitis, and moderate to severe Crohn's disease (CD). In addition, non-systemic corticosteroids (budesonide) have recently become available for the treatment of both CD and UC, demonstrating significant efficacy compared with placebo, with a lower frequency of steroid-related side effects.

Corticosteroids act through a number of different mechanisms. As hormones, they bind to receptors located in the nucleus; the hormone–receptor complex in turn binds to glucocorticoid-responsive elements and activates several transcriptional coactivators, including cAMP response element-binding (CREB) protein, GR-interacting protein (GRP-1) and p300 [1]. These influence several signal transduction pathways that have anti-inflammatory effects by downregulating the inflammatory response through factors such as nuclear factor kappa B (NF-κB) and activator protein 1 (AP1). In addition, glucocorticoids have immunomodulatory effects by acting on white blood cells involved in both the innate and adaptive immune system and reducing the production of proinflammatory agents such as phospholipase A2. Additionally, they may contribute to reduction in the diarrhea associated with both diseases through an effect on the sodium pump.

The initial rate of response to corticosteroid therapy is high, with nearly 90% of patients experiencing some benefit. However, up to one-fifth of patients may develop steroid resistance. The exact mechanism of steroid resistance is unclear but

*Inflammatory Bowel Diseases: A Clinician's Guide*, First Edition. Ashwin N. Ananthakrishnan, Ramnik J. Xavier, and Daniel K. Podolsky.
© 2017 John Wiley & Sons Ltd. Published 2017 by John Wiley & Sons Ltd.

may involve the glucocorticoid receptor, receptor–glucocorticoid responsive element complex, and proteins involved in the extrusion of glucocorticoids from the cell. Patients with steroid-resistant inflammatory bowel disease (IBD) demonstrate lower expression of the glucocorticoid response element mRNA in intestinal mucosa [2]. Genetic polypmorphisms in the tumor necrosis factor (TNF) locus (TNF-α-G308A) [3] and multidrug resistance gene (MDR1) locus are more common in those with steroid resistance and may somehow contribute to its emergence [1]. Circulating lymphocytes and epithelial cells in patients with glucocorticoid-resistant IBD demonstrate greater expression of the P-glycoprotein involved in the extrusion of glucocorticoids from the cell.

## Efficacy in Ulcerative Colitis

Truelove and Witts published a landmark trial establishing the efficacy of corticosteroids in UC in 1955 [4]. In this pivotal study, 210 patients were randomized to receive cortisone or placebo. After 6 weeks, 41% of patients treated with cortisone achieved remission and an additional 28% experienced partial response. A subsequent study demonstrated that prednisone 5 mg four times daily administered in conjunction with 100 mg

hydrocortisone enema daily was more effective than sulfasalazine in achieving remission at 2 weeks (76% vs. 52%) [5]. A dose-ranging study by Baron *et al.* showed that at 5 weeks, remission occurred in two-thirds of patients randomized to 40 or 60 mg of prednisone daily but only in one-third treated with 20 mg per day, establishing a 40 or 60 mg daily dose as the starting dose for the treatment of most flares of moderate to severe UC [6]. There has been no demonstrative benefit to doses of steroids greater than 60 mg per day of prednisone, and higher doses may significantly increase the risk of adverse effects [7]. A population-based study by the Mayo Clinic examined outcomes of 185 patients initiated on systemic corticosteroid therapy between 1970 and 1993 [8]. One year following treatment, fewer than half of the patients (49%) maintained prolonged response despite an 84% rate of complete or partial remission on initiating treatment. More concerning, 22% of patients were steroid dependent and 29% required surgery for management of their disease [8] (Figure 6.1).

Budesonide is an oral corticosteroid that has topical action on the intestine with minimal systemic effect due to a nearly 90% first-pass metabolism in the liver to metabolites with low systemic effects. Ileal release formulations of budesonide have long been available for the management of CD but

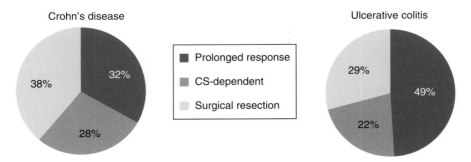

**Figure 6.1** One-year outcomes after initiation of systemic corticosteroid therapy in Crohn's disease and ulcerative colitis. CS, corticosteroid. *Source:* Adapted from Faubion *et al.* 2001 [8]. Reproduced with permission of Elsevier.

were not appropriate for use in UC owing to minimal release in the left colon. A relatively new formulation of budesonide, budesonide MMX®, uses a multi-matrix system technology to release budesonide through the entire colon and has demonstrated efficacy in UC in two randomized controlled trials (RCTs). In the 8-week CORE I clinical trial, both budesonide MMX arms with either a 6 or 9 mg per day dose had greater rates of response than placebo and were similar in efficacy to mesalamine 2.4 g per day [9]. The CORE II trial confirmed this efficacy and also demonstrated improvement in endoscopic and histologic outcomes compared with placebo [10]. Although the mean morning cortisol level was reduced by 103 nmol $l^{-1}$ in the budesonide arm compared with an increase of 28 nmol $l^{-1}$ in the placebo arm, clinically relevant steroid-related adverse events were uncommon and similar between the treatment and placebo arms [10].

Corticosteroids play a particularly important role in the management of acute severe UC requiring hospitalization. They are usually administered intravenously either as hydrocortisone (300–400 mg per day, administered in three or four divided doses or as a continuous drip) or prednisone (40–60 mg per day). Initial trials using 400 mg per day of cortisone in conjunction with rectal enema therapy demonstrated complete remission in 64% of patients, partial response in 13% and failure of treatment in 23% resulting in urgent colectomy [11]. There does not seem to be a dose–response relationship at dosages greater than 60 mg per day of prednisone (48 mg per day of methylprednisolone). Bolus dosing is equivalent to continuous infusion. Intravenous adrenocorticotropic hormone (ACTH) also has similar efficacy and may have a small advantage in steroid-naive patients; however, potential risk of adrenal hemorrhage has limited its use [12]. It is not suitable for patients who have already been receiving corticosteroids in whom adrenal suppression should be assumed.

Topical corticosteroids are available as suppositories (hydrocortisone 25–30 mg daily), foams (cortifoam 80 mg daily, budesonide 2 mg once or twice daily), and enemas (hydrocortisone enemas 100 mg once or twice daily) reaching progressively higher up in the rectum, sigmoid colon, and left colon, respectively. They are effective as initial therapy in the management of mild to moderate distal colitis but they may actually be less effective than topical mesalamine. However, patients with severe disease sometimes tolerate topical corticosteroids better than topical mesalamine, and topical steroids are particularly helpful in those with hypersensitivity to aminosalicylates. The foam or suppository form may be better tolerated that enema in settings where frequency of bowel movements or urgency precludes the retention of enemas. Systemic absorption of topical corticosteroids may be as high as 40–75%; hence topical steroids may not be appropriate long-term agents. Budesonide foam is an alternative that has recently become available.

## Efficacy in Crohn's Disease

Oral corticosteroids are used for the induction of remission in mild to moderate CD. In the National Cooperative Crohn's Disease Study (NCCDS) trial, by week 5 nearly 65% of patients treated with prednisone achieved a Crohn's disease activity index (CDAI) below 150 (considered clinical remission) on at least one occasion, significantly higher than the rates seen with sulfasalazine, azathioprine, or placebo. The European Cooperative Crohn's Disease Study (ECCDS) demonstrated similar efficacy of prednisone in inducing remission in CD. The dose is similar to that in UC, typically up to 40 mg per day. In RCTs, prednisone yielded superior remission rates compared with sulfasalazine, elemental diet, and antibiotics. After achieving remission, tapering of steroids requires judgment by the treating physician. In common practice, the dose is reduced by 5–10 mg per day each week until a level of 20 mg per day is achieved, after which the taper is by 2.5–5 mg per day each week. Similarly to that observed in UC, prolonged response to steroids was seen in only one-third (32%) of patients with CD. Nearly two-thirds developed either corticosteroid dependence or required surgery for management of their disease [8] (Figure 6.1).

Ileal-release budesonide (Entocort®, Budenofalk®) is an attractive alternative for the management of CD involving the ileum or right colon owing to its high topical inflammatory activity and low systemic effect because of high first-pass metabolism. Greenberg *et al.* randomized 258 patients with active CD to placebo or three doses of budesonide (3, 9, or 15 mg per day). At the end of the 8-week study, remission occurred in 51% of patients in the 9 mg budesonide arm, compared with 20% of those receiving placebo [13]. The efficacy of the 15 mg budesonide arm (43%) was lower than that of the 9 mg arm. Although budesonide suppressed basal plasma cortisol, clinically significant steroid-related symptoms were uncommon. A second study, by Rutgeerts *et al.* [14], compared budesonide 9 mg per day with prednisolone beginning at 40 mg per day and tapering over a 10-week period.

At the end of the study, 53% of patients in the budesonide-treated arm were in remission, which was similar to the 66% in those treated with prednisolone. However, the mean reduction in CDAI was greater in the prednisolone than the budesonide arm. A similar result was observed in children [15].

Budesonide has been examined for maintenance of remission. In doses of 6 mg per day, budesonide use was associated with a longer time to relapse or discontinuation of therapy, but the absolute rate of relapse at 1 year was similar to placebo, suggesting lack of effect as a maintenance agent in CD [16].

## Safety

Corticosteroid-related side effects are common and nearly any organ system can be affected (Table 6.1). Most side effects are dose dependent, some are reversible, and some are preventable with appropriate supplementation. There is also considerable heterogeneity in susceptibility to steroid-related side effects. Common side effects include infections, diabetes or impaired glucose tolerance, cataract, glaucoma, hypertension, fluid retention, cushingoid habitus, mood and psychiatric disturbances, sleep disturbances, impaired bone mineralization, and osteonecrosis of the femoral head.

**Table 6.1** Side effects of systemic corticosteroids.

| Organ system | Adverse effect |
| --- | --- |
| Ophthalmologic | Cataract, glaucoma |
| Endocrine | Adrenal suppression, hyperglycemia (diabetes), steroid dependence |
| Musculoskeletal | Osteoporosis, avascular necrosis, myopathy, growth retardation |
| Dermatologic | Acne, moon facies, dermal atrophy, delayed healing |
| Gastrointestinal | Peptic ulcer, pancreatitis |
| Neuropsychiatric | Mood changes, psychosis |
| Cardiovascular | Sodium and water retention, hyperlipidemia |
| Immunologic | Increased susceptibility to infections |

The risk of infections appears greater than that observed with immunomodulator or biologic treatment, and steroids may confer an additive increase in infection risk in patients on immunosuppressive therapy [17]. To minimize the effect on bone mineral density, the use of steroids should be accompanied by concomitant supplementation with calcium (1–2 g per day) and vitamin D (1000 IU daily). Patients who are on significant doses of systemic steroids for at least 3 months should undergo a dual-energy X-ray absorptiometry (DEXA) scan to screen for osteopenia. Osteonecrosis of the femoral head is usually irreversible and sometimes requires hip replacement for relief of pain and restoration of joint function. Patients on long-term corticosteroids should also undergo periodic ophthalmologic evaluations for diagnosis of glaucoma and posterior subcapsular cataracts. Monitoring for steroid-related side effects should also be performed with the use of agents such as budesonide despite its high first-pass metabolism and lower systemic effects. In the budesonide maintenance trials, corticosteroid-related adverse effects occurred in fewer patients in the budesonide than in the prednisolone arm ($p = 0.003$). Given the range and severity of side effects, steroids should be used at the lowest dose for the shortest possible duration.

# Case Studies and Multiple Choice Questions

1  Which of the following statements are *not* true regarding the use of budesonide in the management of Crohn's disease?
   A  Budesonide is not effective for maintenance of remission in Crohn's disease at 1 year.
   B  It is associated with a similar degree of adrenal suppression and steroid-related side effects as prednisone.
   C  Budesonide (Entocort®) is effective for induction of remission in ileal and right colonic Crohn's disease.

2  Which of the following side effects are *not* seen with corticosteroid therapy?
   A  Increased risk of skin cancer.
   B  Osteonecrosis of the femoral head.
   C  Glaucoma.
   D  Mood disturbances.

3  Corinne is a 19-year-old woman with ulcerative colitis hospitalized with 10 bowel movements per day, most of which contain blood. She has received 5 days of treatment with intravenous steroids in the form of methylprednisolone 20 mg every 8 h with no improvement in her symptoms. Which of the following would be the best next step in her management?
   A  Increase the methylprednisolone dose to 40 mg every 8 h.
   B  Increase the methylprednisolone dose to 1 g daily and add topical hydrocortisone enemas.
   C  Initiate therapy with azathioprine.
   D  Initiate therapy with infliximab.

# References

1 De Iudicibus, S., Franca, R., Martelossi, S., *et al.* (2011) Molecular mechanism of glucocorticoid resistance in inflammatory bowel disease. *World Journal of Gastroenterology*, **17**(9), 1095–1108.

2 Raddatz, D., Middel, P., Bockemühl, M., *et al.* (2004) Glucocorticoid receptor expression in inflammatory bowel disease: evidence for a mucosal down-regulation in steroid-unresponsive ulcerative colitis. *Alimentary Pharmacology & Therapeutics*, **19**(1), 47–61.

3 Cucchiara, S., Latiano, A., Palmieri, O., *et al.* (2007) Polymorphisms of tumor necrosis factor-alpha but not MDR1 influence response to medical therapy in pediatric-onset inflammatory bowel disease. *Journal of Pediatric Gastroenterology and Nutrition*, **44**(2), 171–179.

4 Truelove, S.C. and Witts, L.J. (1955) Cortisone in ulcerative colitis; final report on a therapeutic trial. *British Medical Journal*, **ii**(4947), 1041–1048.

5 Truelove, S.C., Watkinson, G., and Draper, G. (1962) Comparison of corticosteroid and sulphasalazine therapy in ulcerative colitis. *British Medical Journal*, **ii**(5321), 1708–1711.

6 Baron, J.H., Connell, A.M., Kanaghinis, T.G., *et al.* (1962) Out-patient treatment of ulcerative colitis. Comparison between three doses of oral prednisone. *British Medical Journal*, **ii**(5302), 441–443.

7 Turner, D., Walsh, C.M., Steinhart, A.H., and Griffiths, A.M. (2007) Response to corticosteroids in severe ulcerative colitis: a systematic review of the literature and a meta-regression. *Clinical Gastroenterology and Hepatology*, **5**(1), 103–110.

8 Faubion,W.A., Jr., Loftus, E.V., Jr., Harmsen, W.S., *et al.* (2001) The natural history of corticosteroid therapy for inflammatory bowel disease: a population-based study. *Gastroenterology*, **121**(2), 255–260.

9 Sandborn, W.J., Travis, S., Moro, L., *et al.* (2012) Once-daily budesonide MMX® extended-release tablets induce remission in patients with mild to moderate ulcerative colitis: results from the CORE I study. *Gastroenterology*, **143**(5), 1218–1226.e2.

10 Travis, S.P.L., Danese, S., Kupcinskas, L., *et al.* (2014) Once-daily budesonide MMX in active, mild-to-moderate ulcerative colitis: results from the randomised CORE II study. *Gut*, **63**(3), 433–441.

11 Truelove, S.C. and Jewell, D.P. (1974) Intensive intravenous regimen for severe attacks of ulcerative colitis. *Lancet*, **i**(7866), 1067–1070.

12 Kaplan, H.P., Portnoy, B., Binder, H.J., *et al.* (1975) A controlled evaluation of intravenous adrenocorticotropic hormone and hydrocortisone in the treatment of acute colitis. *Gastroenterology*, **69**(1), 91–95.

13 Greenberg, G.R., Feagan, B.G., Martin, F., *et al.* (1994) Oral budesonide for active Crohn's disease. Canadian Inflammatory Bowel Disease Study Group. *New England Journal of Medicine*, **331**(13), 836–841.

14 Rutgeerts, P., Löfberg, R., Malchow, H., *et al.* (1994) A comparison of budesonide with prednisolone for active Crohn's disease. *New England Journal of Medicine*, **331**(13), 842–845.

15 Escher, J.C. and European Collaborative Research Group on Budesonide in Paediatric IBD (2004) Budesonide versus prednisolone for the treatment of active Crohn's disease in children: a randomized, double-blind, controlled, multicentre trial. *European Journal of Gastroenterology & Hepatology*, **16**(1), 47–54.

16 Greenberg, G.R., Feagan, B.G., Martin, F., *et al.* (1996) Oral budesonide as maintenance treatment for Crohn's disease: a placebo-controlled, dose-ranging study. Canadian Inflammatory Bowel Disease Study Group. *Gastroenterology*, **110**(1), 45–51.

17 Toruner, M., Loftus, E.V., Jr., Harmsen, W.S., *et al.* (2008) Risk factors for opportunistic infections in patients with inflammatory bowel disease. *Gastroenterology*, **134**(4), 929–936.

## Answers to Questions

1 Answer: **B**. Although budesonide suppresses basal plasma cortisol in clinical trials, clinically significant steroid-related symptoms are uncommon. At a dose of 6 mg per day, budesonide use was associated with a longer time to relapse, but the absolute rate of relapse at 1 year was similar to that with placebo, suggesting a lack of effect as a maintenance agent in CD [16].

2 Answer: **A**. Common side effects include infections, impaired glucose tolerance, cataract, glaucoma, hypertension, fluid retention, cushingoid habitus, mood and psychiatric disturbances, sleep disturbances, impaired bone mineralization and osteonecrosis of the femoral head.

Immunosuppression-related malignancies including skin cancers and lymphoma have not been reported with corticosteroid therapy.

3 Answer: **D**. Corinne has acute severe ulcerative colitis refractory to corticosteroids. There does not appear to be a dose–response relationship beyond 60 mg per day of methylprednisolone, so increasing the dose to 120 mg or 1 g daily is not likely to result in benefit and will increase the risk of adverse outcomes. Azathioprine is not effective in induction of remission in steroid-refractory ulcerative colitis, so initiation of infliximab is the best next step in her care.

# 7

# Immunomodulators

---

## Clinical Take Home Messages

- Thiopurines are not effective for inducing remission in Crohn's disease or ulcerative colitis owing to delayed onset of action. They can be effective in maintaining remission in moderate to severe disease
- Idiosyncratic and dose-related adverse events are common with thiopurine use. All patients should have a thiopurine methyltransferase enzyme level or genotype checked prior to initiation of thiopurine therapy.
- Measurements of thiopurine metabolite levels (6-thioguanine, 6-methylmercaptopurine) are useful to guide optimizing dosing in the setting of non-response confirmed by objective evidence of active inflammation. Addition of allopurinol may result in therapeutic efficacy in a subset of patients who otherwise shunt 6-mercaptopurine production towards 6-methylmercaptopurine rather than 6-thioguanine.
- Thiopurines are associated with an increased risk of infections, non-melanoma skin cancers, and lymphoma.
- Methotrexate has been demonstrated to be effective in the treatment of Crohn's disease when administered parenterally. Oral methotrexate is ineffective as monotherapy in ulcerative colitis.
- Cyclosporine is effective in inducing remission in steroid-refractory ulcerative colitis.

---

Immunomodulators or immunosuppressants exert their effect through modification of systemic immune responses. The commonly used immunomodulators include thiopurines (azathioprine, 6-mercaptopurine), other antimetabolites (methotrexate), and calcineurin inhibitors (cyclosporine, tacrolimus). They are traditionally used in patients who are steroid dependent or steroid refractory

## Thiopurines

Azathioprine is a prodrug that undergoes initial conversion to 6-mercaptopurine (6-MP), its active form (Figure 7.1). 6-MP is converted through a series of steps catalyzed by the enzyme thiopurine methyltransferase (TPMT) to 6-thioguanine (6-TGN), which represents its active metabolite, and 6-methylmercaptopurine (6-MMP), a

*Inflammatory Bowel Diseases: A Clinician's Guide,* First Edition. Ashwin N. Ananthakrishnan, Ramnik J. Xavier, and Daniel K. Podolsky.
© 2017 John Wiley & Sons Ltd. Published 2017 by John Wiley & Sons Ltd.

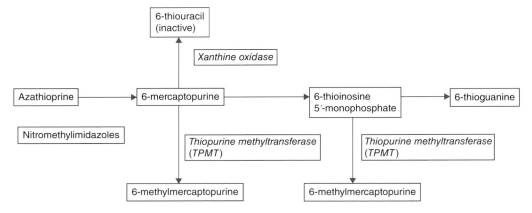

**Figure 7.1** Metabolism of thiopurines.

hepatotoxic agent. Knowledge of the metabolism of thiopurine is essential for understanding the role of metabolite monitoring in the setting of adverse effects such as hepatotoxicity, and lack of efficacy, as well as to interaction with other therapies (such as aminosalicylates and allopurinol). Several mechanisms explain the efficacy of thiopurines in inflammatory bowel disease (IBD) and other immune-mediated diseases. As an anti-metabolite, the 6-TGN accumulates intracellularly, inhibiting purine metabolism, and consequently DNA synthesis and cell proliferation. Thiopurines may also act directly on lymphocytes, plasma cells, and natural killer cells.

There is considerable heterogeneity in the activity of the TPMT enzyme. Approximately 88% of the population carries the wild-type TPMT allele, which is associated with normal enzyme activity and normal metabolism of thiopurines. An estimated 11% carry a variant allele associated with an intermediate level of enzyme activity, and a propensity to generate higher levels of 6-TGN metabolites resulting in superior efficacy but also a higher risk of leukopenia. Importantly, 0.3% of patients carry two variant alleles of the TPMT gene, resulting in low or absent enzyme activity. Such patients are at a high risk for leukopenia with even low doses of

thiopurines and their use is usually contraindicated in such individuals. However, the level of TPMT enzyme activity itself does not appear to influence therapeutic efficacy [1], and the frequency distribution of the various TPMT enzyme phenotypes vary between different populations [2]. TPMT enzyme activity can either be determined by direct measurement of the enzyme activity or inferred by TPMT genotype testing. Both are widely available and routinely used in clinical practice. Either one of these tests is sufficient and should be performed prior to initiating thiopurine therapy. Ongoing thiopurine treatment or use of aminosalicylates may induce TPMT enzyme activity, leading to falsely elevated TMPT levels. In patients with normal TPMT activity, the target dose to achieve adequate therapeutic efficacy is $2.0$–$2.5$ mg kg$^{-1}$ of azathioprine (AZA) or $1.0$–$1.5$ mg kg$^{-1}$ of 6-MP. However, some patients may require doses as high as $3.0$–$3.5$ mg kg$^{-1}$ of AZA to achieve the optimal therapeutic concentration. Most patients are initiated on 1 mg kg$^{-1}$ of AZA or equivalent dose of 6-MP and titrated up to their target dose over the next few weeks. One reason for beginning therapy with low doses of thiopurines is that most cases of leukopenia occur in patients with normal TPMT activity. Complete blood

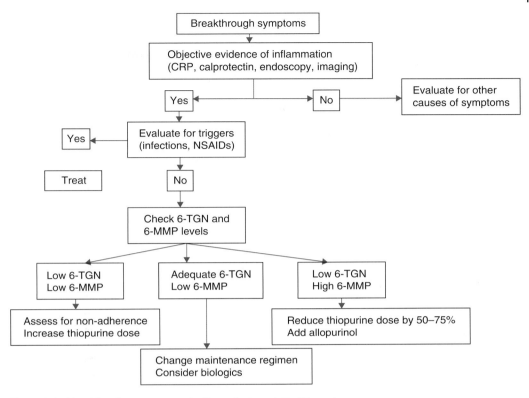

**Figure 7.2** Algorithm for management of loss of response to thiopurines.

counts and liver enzymes are monitored every 2–3 weeks after initiating AZA/6-MP, and the dose is escalated to target with each normal laboratory test. Once the patient has reached a stable dose, monitoring frequency can be reduced to every 3–4 months.

In patients who fail to respond or lose an initial response to thiopurine therapy, measurement of thiopurine metabolite levels (both 6-TGN and 6-MMP) may have a role in therapeutic decision-making (Figure 7.2). In retrospective studies, 6-TGN levels above 235–250 pmol per $8 \times 10^8$ erythrocytes have been associated with greater rates of response. In a study of 92 pediatric patients, the frequency of therapeutic response in those with levels above this threshold was 78% compared to 41% in patients with levels below 235 pmol per $8 \times 10^8$ erythrocytes [3].

However, such an association has not been confirmed in all cohorts [4]. Measurement of metabolite levels can also identify the subgroup of patients who preferentially shunt 6-MP metabolism towards the 6-MMP pathway. Coadministration of low-dose allopurinol by reversing this shunt can produce durable remission [5]. However, it is important to undertake more frequent blood count monitoring in such patients to avoid toxicity due to the potentially marked increase in 6-TGN.

**Efficacy in Ulcerative Colitis**

Owing to the long time lag between therapy initiation and effect, thiopurines are not useful for the induction of remission in ulcerative colitis (UC). Despite widespread use, few randomized controlled trials (RCTs) exist in which their role in the maintenance of remission in UC was examined. Jewell and Truelove first reported the results of a therapeutic trial of AZA in 40 patients randomized to treatment or placebo [6]. As all patients were enrolled in a state of active disease, not surprisingly there was no difference in the initial outcomes. However, at 1 year, there was a strong trend towards higher rates of relapse-free survival in the AZA arm (38%) compared with placebo (12%). A Cochrane review summarized six studies comparing AZA with placebo and concluded that 44% of patients treated with AZA failed to maintain remission compared with 65% with placebo [7]. Two small unblinded trials compared AZA or 6-MP with sulfasalazine or mesalamine [7]. In the trial by Sood *et al.*, 58% of patients treated with AZA failed to maintain remission compared with 38% of patients treated with sulfasalazine [8]. In contrast, Maté-Jiménez *et al.* found a relapse rate of 50% in patients treated with 6-MP compared with 100% in those treated with mesalamine [9]. A single trial by Maté-Jiménez *et al.* compared 6-MP with methotrexate and demonstrated similar efficacy in maintaining remission in steroid-dependent IBD [9].

Some clinical trials have adopted the approach of therapy withdrawal to determine the efficacy of maintenance therapy [10, 11]. In a study of 79 patients on AZA for 6 months or more, most of whom had been in full remission for 2 months or more, 36% of patients continuing therapy relapsed at 1 year compared with 59% of those administered placebo [10]. This benefit was seen even in those who had been in long-term remission. Lack of sustained remission, extensive colitis, and short treatment duration were associated with higher rates of relapse and concomitant therapy with aminosalicylates was protective against relapses [11]. Observational cohorts have demonstrated sustained efficacy of AZA in UC. In a study of 622 patients treated with AZA,

the proportion remaining in remission at 1, 3, and 5 years was 0.95, 0.69, and 0.55, respectively [12]. Similar long-term outcomes have been reported with 6-MP treatment [13].

Some groups have proposed the use of 6-TGN, the active metabolite itself, as a therapeutic agent, particularly in patients who are resistant or intolerant to 6-MP. In a small series of 16 patients, a complete response was observed in 36% and a partial response in 43% of subjects [14]. However, the risk of nodular regenerative hyperplasia limits the use of 6-TGN. Intravenous AZA was examined in a small study consisting of nine patients with steroid-refractory UC and demonstrated response in 56% of the patients [15].

## Efficacy in Crohn's Disease

Several RCTs have examined the efficacy of AZA and 6-MP in inducing and maintaining remission in CD. In a meta-analysis of 13 RCTs and 1211 patients with active CD treated with AZA, 6-MP, or placebo, there was no difference in clinical remission or response rates between AZA or 6-MP and placebo [16]. However, 64% of patients treated with AZA were able to reduce their dose to ≤10 mg per day of prednisone compared with 46% of those treated with placebo [16].

In contrast, AZA may indeed have a role in the maintenance of remission. Candy *et al.* performed a landmark trial, randomizing 63 patients with active CD treated with prednisolone to receive AZA or placebo [17]. Over a 15-month follow-up, a larger proportion of patients in the AZA arm were in remission (42%) than those who received placebo (7%). Clinical response was accompanied by a reduction in C-reactive protein, erythrocyte sedimentation rate, and leukocyte count in the AZA group. Markowitz *et al.* demonstrated similar efficacy and lower cumulative steroid dose with the use of 6-MP in newly diagnosed CD [18] A meta-analysis of five trials identified an overall remission rate of 71% with AZA compared with 55% for placebo with a corresponding number needed to treat of 6. Similarly to that observed in UC, withdrawal of AZA in patients in long-term remission is associated with an increased risk of relapse, even in patients who have been in clinical remission for 5 years or longer [19–21]. Despite these previous findings, two recent trials have called the efficacy of AZA in CD into question. Panes *et al.* randomized patients within 8 weeks of diagnosis to AZA 2.5 mg kg$^{-1}$ or placebo. After 76 weeks of treatment, the rates of sustained corticosteroid-free remission were similar between the two groups. However, the relapse rate, defined as a Crohn's disease activity index (CDAI) greater than 220, was lower in the AZA group than the placebo group [22]. A second RCT of early AZA administration compared with conventional management with step-up therapy found no difference in efficacy during the 3-year follow-up but identified a reduced need for perianal surgery [23].

AZA has also been examined in fistulizing perianal CD. In an open-label study, patients who received AZA were more likely to achieve a treatment response in combination with 8 weeks of ciprofloxacin and metronidazole (48%) compared with those on no immunosuppression (15%). After 3 years of therapy, the cumulative probability of remaining free of perianal complications was 47% with AZA or 6-MP use. Shorter duration of perianal disease and older age were predictive of response [24]. Intravenous AZA has not been shown to be effective in the treatment of CD.

### Safety

Adverse effects are common in thiopurine users and are a reason for cessation of therapy in 5–10% of patients. Some adverse events, such as leukopenia or hepatotoxicity, may be dose related whereas others, such as pancreatitis, are independent of the dose. Some side effects are common to both AZA and 6-MP, whereas others that occur with AZA may not recur on rechallenging with 6-MP, which is usually tolerated better. Common adverse effects after initiation include nausea and gastrointestinal side effects, hepatitis, pancreatitis, and infections. Malignancy is a more rare complication. Pancreatitis may occur in up to 5% of patients initiating thiopurines and represents an idiosyncratic reaction not related to TPMT enzyme activity or dose of therapy [25]. Although case reports suggested that 6-MP may be safely initiated in some patients with AZA-induced pancreatitis [26], such reports are few and far between and pancreatitis with one thiopurine agent remains a relative contraindication for rechallenge with another thiopurine. Pancytopenias may occur with thiopurines, although leukopenia is most common. This is usually dose related and responds to a dose reduction. Although intermediate or low TPMT enzyme activity is associated with a higher risk of leukopenia, most patients with thiopurine-induced leukopenia have a normal TPMT enzyme activity [27]. Leukopenia can occur as long as 87 months after initiation of therapy in patients with normal TPMT enzyme activity, suggesting a need for continued complete blood count monitoring.

Hepatotoxicity is another common adverse effect related to thiopurine metabolism. It is thought to result from elevated 6-MMP concentrations (above 5700 pmol per $8 \times 10^8$ erythrocytes). Development of such elevated 6-MMP levels in combination with subtherapeutic 6-TGN concentrations is seen in a subgroup of patients who shunt thiopurine metabolism preferentially towards 6-MMP formation. The reason for this shunting is unclear, but the use of low-dose allopurinol in conjunction with a reduction in the dose of thiopurines usually reverses the phenomenon, and restores 6-TGN values to therapeutic levels while reducing the concentration of 6-MMP [28, 29]. Other hepatotoxic effects of thiopurines include cholestatic hepatitis, nodular regenerative hyperplasia, and veno-occlusive disease.

Infections are more common in patients receiving AZA compared with placebo, but rates are lower than with corticosteroid therapy [30]. Although infections may occur in 6–7% of patients with AZA-induced leukopenia, most infections occur in the absence of leukopenia. AZA/6-MP also confers a threefold increase in the risk of opportunistic infections [30].

Treatment-related malignancies, particularly lymphoma and skin cancers, are an important concern with long-term immunosuppressive therapy. Compared with non-users, current thiopurine use is associated with an up to fourfold increase in risk of lymphoma, primarily non-Hodgkin's lymphoma (NHL) [31]. The incidence may increase with successively longer duration of use from <1 year to >4 years, and reduce or return to normal after cessation of therapy [32]. The absolute risk of NHL among thiopurine users ranges from 4 to 6 per 10 000 patient-years compared with 1.9 per 10 000 person-years in the control population. A rare form of aggressive lymphoma, hepatosplenic T-cell lymphoma (HSTCL), has been associated both with thiopurine monotherapy and their use in conjunction with biologics [33]. In a series of 36 patients with HSTCL, 20 were treated with combination therapy and 16 had received thiopurine monotherapy. Nearly all of the patients were men and younger than 35 years of age, suggesting an increased absolute risk in this cohort.

Studies of several cohorts in North America and Europe have demonstrated an increase in risk for non-melanoma skin cancers in both current and past users of thiopurines [34, 35]. The increase in risk appears to be more modest for basal cell carcinoma than squamous cell cancer. In a study by Long *et al.*, thiopurine use was associated with increased risk of non-melanoma skin cancers but not melanoma [35]. There appears to be no increase in risk of solid organ tumors with thiopurine use. In a large series of 2204 patients, 626 were treated with thiopurine and the overall risk of cancer (4.5% in each group) and colorectal neoplasms (2.2% vs. 2.8%) was similar between thiopurine users and non-users [36].

## Methotrexate

Methotrexate is an antimetabolite that exerts its effect through competitive inhibition of dihydrofolate reductase and interference with purine production and DNA synthesis. The bioavailability of intramuscular or subcutaneously administered methotrexate is as high as 90%; however, oral administration results in variable lower bioavailability. Both parenteral and oral methotrexate have been studied in IBD, with only the parenteral formulation demonstrating efficacy in clinical trials.

### Efficacy in Ulcerative Colitis

Only one RCT has examined the efficacy of methotrexate in UC [37]. Oren *et al.* randomized 67 patients to 12.5 mg of oral methotrexate once per week or placebo for 9 months. At the end of the trial, the proportion of patients in remission was 47% in the methotrexate arm, nearly identical with 49% in the placebo arm. The proportion of patients relapsing and the mean steroid dose were also similar in both groups. Whether this represents lack of efficacy of methotrexate in UC or was due to variable oral bioavailability and under-dosing is unclear. The ongoing Methotrexate in Induction and Maintenance of Steroid Free Remission in Ulcerative Colitis (MERIT-UC) study may provide additional information regarding its efficacy in UC. Open-label observational studies suggest that methotrexate, when administered parenterally and at a higher dose, was able to maintain steroid-free remission at the end of two years in 35% of thiopurine-failed patients [38].

### Efficacy in Crohn's Disease

In contrast to the lack of data supporting the efficacy of methotrexate in UC, RCT data support its efficacy in CD. A double-blind placebo-controlled trial randomized 141 patients with active CD to methotrexate or placebo. At the end of 16 weeks of this induction trial, 39% of patients in the methotrexate group were in clinical remission compared with 19% of patients on placebo [39]. The total dose of steroids was also lower in methotrexate users. In the maintenance phase of the trial utilizing 15 mg of intramuscular methotrexate weekly, 65% of patients in the methotrexate group were in remission at the end of the study compared with 14% of those treated with placebo [40]. However, in a subsequent study of patients with CD initiating prednisone treatment, a combination of methotrexate and infliximab was similar in efficacy to infliximab monotherapy [41]. Observational cohorts confirm the efficacy of methotrexate in CD, including in thiopurine non-responders and patients with perianal disease [42, 43].

### Safety

Owing to its mechanism of action, methotrexate is associated with folate deficiency and users must also take supplemental folate at a dose of 1 mg per day. Long-term methotrexate use is associated with several side effects, primarily hepatotoxicity. A systematic review of patients with rheumatoid arthritis found that 13% of methotrexate users had an elevation of their liver enzymes and 4% stopped therapy owing to hepatotoxicity. Significant fibrosis and cirrhosis can be seen in 2–33% and 0–26% of patients, respectively, with long-term methotrexate use [44]. This hepatotoxicity is related to cumulative dose, although genetic polymorphisms may also influence susceptibility [45]. As hepatic fibrosis may not always manifest as elevated liver enzymes, some recommend liver biopsy after every cumulative dose of 1.5 g of methotrexate. However, recent guidelines suggest that such practice may be unnecessary with careful monitoring. An unexplained or persistent decrease in serum albumin in long-term methotrexate users should raise suspicion for potential hepatotoxicity. Methotrexate is a well-known teratogen. Its use in women in the reproductive age group should be accompanied by appropriate birth control precautions. Although paternal exposure has not been associated with congenital abnormalities, therapy is usually stopped at least 3–6 months prior to conception in both men and women. Pulmonary fibrosis is also a well-known side effect of methotrexate.

## Calcineurin Inhibitors

Both cyclosporine and tacrolimus exert their effects by binding to and inhibiting calcineurin, an enzyme required for activation of T-lymphocytes. Cyclosporine is used more commonly than tacrolimus, although the use of both is infrequent and limited to specialized centers. Each is associated with significant potential for toxicity and close monitoring of blood levels is required.

### Efficacy in Ulcerative Colitis

Cyclosporine is usually administered in the setting of acute severe steroid-refractory colitis in hospitalized patients. It is administered intravenously in doses of 2–4 mg kg$^{-1}$ with dose titration to achieve optimal serum concentrations of 250–400 ng ml$^{-1}$. The onset of action of cyclosporine is rapid, usually within a few days. Patients who respond to the intravenous cyclosporine are converted to oral cyclosporine. The bioavailability of oral cyclosporine is lower than that with the intravenous formulation, and conversion to oral therapy usually requires a twofold increase in dose. Continuation of cyclosporine without addition of a concomitant maintenance immunomodulator agent is associated with higher rates of treatment failure and colectomy. In a 5-year follow-up of 42 patients who received intravenous cyclosporine, 20% of those who received AZA or 6-MP required colectomy compared with 45% of those not receiving either of these therapies [46]. Oral cyclosporine is maintained for a period of 3–6 months, after which the immunomodulator is continued as the sole therapy. Serum levels of cyclosporine should be obtained twice per week until a stable oral dose has been achieved, after which weekly laboratory testing is sufficient. Serum levels of magnesium and a lipid panel must be obtained prior to initiation of cyclosporine as its use has been associated with seizures in the setting of low levels of either magnesium or cholesterol. Nephrotoxicity is a common dose-related adverse effect of cyclosporine, necessitating frequent monitoring of renal function. A reduction in creatinine clearance of ≥20% may occur. Neurologic side effects including headaches and paresthesias also occur occasionally and respond to reduction in dose or cessation of therapy. Infections are a serious complication that can occur with cyclosporine, particularly as patients are ill, malnourished, and often on concomitant therapy with corticosteroids and immunomodulators. Hence many providers frequently administer prophylaxis against *Pneumocystis jiroveci* pneumonia.

Lichtiger *et al.* performed a landmark RCT establishing the efficacy of cyclosporine in the management of acute steroid-refractory UC in an era when there were few other options for avoiding colectomy in this cohort [47]. Although the trial included only 20 patients, the results were striking. Nine out of 11 patients treated with intravenous cyclosporine 4 mg kg$^{-1}$ responded, compared with none of the patients treated with placebo. Five patients in the placebo group were subsequently treated with cyclosporine and all responded. Several subsequent studies demonstrated a comparably high rate of response to intravenous cyclosporine in steroid-refractory colitis [48, 49]. During 3 years of follow-up, 55% of patients avoided colectomy [49]. A Belgian trial compared low-dose (2 mg kg$^{-1}$) with high-dose (4 mg kg$^{-1}$) cyclosporine and demonstrated comparable rates of response at day 8 (84% vs. 86%), although the higher dose was associated with a higher incidence of hypertension [50]. The initial cyclosporine trials were in patients who were refractory to steroids. D'Haens *et al.* randomized patients on hospitalization to either intravenous cyclosporine or methylprednisolone and found similar rates of response in both groups [51]. The place of cyclosporine in the therapeutic management of acute severe colitis has been challenged by the introduction and availability of infliximab. RCTs demonstrated a similar response rate with infliximab (compared with placebo). Moreover, infliximab offers the option of continuing as the maintenance agent in responders without the need to use it solely as a bridge. Until recently, there were few comparative data to guide treatment selection. Laharie *et al.* performed an open-label trial, randomizing 115 patients to treatment with either cyclosporine or infliximab at 27 European centers. Both groups were initiated on AZA therapy [52]. At days 7 and 98, both groups achieved similar rates of response and likelihood of colectomy.

Although intravenous administration of tacrolimus has been used in the management of steroid-refractory colitis, it is more commonly administered orally. Initially dosed at 0.10–0.15 mg kg$^{-1}$, therapy is titrated to achieve trough levels of 10–20 ng ml$^{-1}$. Patients initiated on tacrolimus are also

commonly transitioned to other oral immunomodulator therapies for maintenance.
The efficacy of oral tacrolimus in the management of hospitalized patients with
steroid-refractory colitis was examined in a
double-blind placebo-controlled trial [53].
At week 2, the clinical response rate in the
tacrolimus group was significantly greater
than that in the placebo group (50% vs. 13%),
paralleling a higher rate of mucosal healing
(44% vs. 13%).

### Efficacy in Crohn's Disease

There are limited data supporting the efficacy of cyclosporine in CD. High doses of
oral cyclosporine (5–7.5 mg kg$^{-1}$) are associated with improvement in disease activity but nearly one-third of patients had to
withdraw owing to side effects [54]. A subsequent double-blind RCT of low-dose
cyclosporine in those with active treatment (60%) found no difference in the rate
of relapse compared with placebo (52%)
[55]. Small case series demonstrated
the efficacy of cyclosporine in steroid-
refractory CD, although high-quality data
guiding cyclosporine use in this setting are

lacking [56, 57] and the availability of other
effective therapies limits much of the need
for cyclosporine. It has also been studied
in small series of patients with perianal fistulae, demonstrating good (88–90%) initial
improvement but high rates of relapse in
the absence of maintenance immunomodulator therapy.

The role of tacrolimus in CD is primarily
in fistulizing disease. In a systematic review
including 163 patients, the pooled remission rate with tacrolimus use for luminal
CD was 44%. Most studies were open label
and did not have a placebo arm for comparison. Tacrolimus has been used as a sole
therapy and in combination with AZA or
6-MP for the management of perianal
fistulae with modest efficacy [58]. A randomized placebo-controlled trial in patients
with CD with draining perianal or enterocutaneous fistulae demonstrated a 43%
rate of improvement of perianal fistula by
10 weeks with tacrolimus compared with
8% with placebo [59]. However, side effects
including headache, increased serum
creatinine, paresthesias, and tremor were
common.

# Case Studies and Multiple Choice Questions

1 Which of the following side effects is not commonly seen with thiopurine therapy for Crohn's disease and ulcerative colitis?
   A Pancreatitis.
   B Paradoxical worsening of colitis.
   C Fever, arthralgia, and flu-like symptoms.
   D Increased risk of lymphoma.

2 Alexandra is a 25-year-old woman with ileocecal Crohn's disease, non-stricturing, non-penetrating phenotype, who presents to you for follow-up 5 months after initiation of azathioprine at an appropriate dose of 150 mg daily ($2.5$ mg kg$^{-1}$). She reports that for the past month, she has been having increasing abdominal pain and diarrhea consistent with an exacerbation of her Crohn's disease. She denies missing any doses. You obtain thiopurine metabolite levels. This reveals a 6-TGN level of 135 pmol per $8 \times 10^8$ erythrocytes and a 6-MMPN level of 7500 pmol per $8 \times 10^8$ erythrocytes. Which of the following is an appropriate alteration in her thiopurine regimen?
   A Increase azathioprine to 200 mg daily.
   B Reduce azathioprine to 100 mg daily.
   C Add prednisone 40 mg per day, reduce azathioprine to 50 mg per day, and add allopurinol 100 mg per day.
   D Add prednisone 40 mg per day and continue azathioprine 150 mg per day.

3 Which of the following statements is true about myelosuppression in patients on thiopurine therapy?
   A Most patients who develop low white blood cell (WBC) counts have intermediate or deficient TPMT enzyme activity.
   B Myelosuppression is seen only within the first 3 months of initiation of thiopurine therapy.
   C Most patients who develop myelosuppression have normal TPMT enzyme activity.
   D Elevated levels of 6-MMPN predispose patients to low WBC counts on thiopurine therapy.

4 Which of the following statements about the use of methotrexate in Crohn's disease is true?
   A Oral methotrexate 15 mg weekly is effective for the induction of remission in Crohn's disease.
   B Intramuscular methotrexate 25 mg weekly is effective for the induction of remission in Crohn's disease.
   C There are no data supporting the role of methotrexate in maintaining remission in Crohn's disease.
   D Methotrexate in combination with infliximab was associated with a higher rate of mucosal healing at 1 year than infliximab monotherapy in patients with Crohn's disease.

# References

1 Gonzalez-Lama, Y., Bermejo, F., Lopez-Sanroman, A., *et al.* (2011) Thiopurine methyl-transferase activity and azathioprine metabolite concentrations do not predict clinical outcome in thiopurine-treated inflammatory bowel disease patients. *Alimentary Pharmacology & Therapeutics*, **34**(5), 544–554.

2 Krynetski, E.Y., Tai, H.L., Yates, C.R., *et al.* (1996) Genetic polymorphism of thiopurine *S*-methyltransferase: clinical importance and molecular mechanisms. *Pharmacogenetics*, **6**(4), 279–290.

3 Dubinsky, M.C., Lamothe, S., Yang, H.Y., *et al.* (2000) Pharmacogenomics and metabolite measurement for 6-mercaptopurine therapy in inflammatory bowel disease. *Gastroenterology*, **118**(4), 705–713.

4 Goldenberg, B.A., Rawsthorne, P., and Bernstein, C.N. (2004) The utility of 6-thioguanine metabolite levels in managing patients with inflammatory bowel disease. *American Journal of Gastroenterology*, **99**(9), 1744–1748.

5 Sandborn, W.J., Travis, S., Moro, L., *et al.* (2012) Once-daily budesonide MMX® extended-release tablets induce remission in patients with mild to moderate ulcerative colitis: results from the CORE I study. *Gastroenterology*, **143**(5), 1218–1226.e2.

6 Jewell, D.P., and Truelove, S.C. (1974) Azathioprine in ulcerative colitis: final report on controlled therapeutic trial. *British Medical Journal*, **4**(5945), 627–630.

7 Timmer, A., McDonald, J.W., Tsoulis, D.J., and Macdonald, J.K. (2012) Azathioprine and 6-mercaptopurine for maintenance of remission in ulcerative colitis. *Cochrane Database of Systematic Reviews*, (**9**), CD000478.

8 Sood, A., Midha, V., Sood, N., and Avasthi, G. (2003) Azathioprine versus sulfasalazine in maintenance of remission in severe ulcerative colitis. *Indian Journal of Gastroenterology*, **22**(3), 79–81.

9 Maté-Jiménez, J., Hermida, C., Cantero-Perona, J., and Moreno-Otero, R. (2000) 6-Mercaptopurine or methotrexate added to prednisone induces and maintains remission in steroid-dependent inflammatory bowel disease. *European Journal of Gastroenterology & Hepatology*, **12**(11), 1227–1233.

10 Hawthorne, A.B., Logan, R.F., Hawkey, C.J., *et al.* (1992) Randomised controlled trial of azathioprine withdrawal in ulcerative colitis. *BMJ (Clinical Research Edition)*, **305**(6844), 20–22.

11 Cassinotti, A., Actis, G.C., Duca, P., *et al.* (2009) Maintenance treatment with azathioprine in ulcerative colitis: outcome and predictive factors after drug withdrawal. *American Journal of Gastroenterology*, **104**(11), 2760–2767.

12 Fraser, A.G., Orchard, T.R., and Jewell, D.P. (2002) The efficacy of azathioprine for the treatment of inflammatory bowel disease: a 30 year review. *Gut*, **50**(4), 485–489.

13 George, J., Present, D.H., Pou, R., *et al.* (1996) The long-term outcome of ulcerative colitis treated with 6-mercaptopurine. *American Journal of Gastroenterology*, **91**(9), 1711–1714.

14 Teml, A., Schwab, M., Harrer, M., *et al.* (2005) A prospective, open-label trial of 6-thioguanine in patients with ulcerative or indeterminate colitis. *Scandinavian Journal of Gastroenterology*, **40**(10), 1205–1213.

15 Mahadevan, U., Tremaine, W.J., Johnson, T., *et al.* (2000) Intravenous azathioprine in severe ulcerative colitis: a pilot study. *American Journal of Gastroenterology*, **95**(12), 3463–3468.

16 Chande, N., Tsoulis, D.J., and MacDonald, J.K. (2013) Azathioprine or 6-mercaptopurine for induction of remission in Crohn's disease. *Cochrane Database of Systematic Reviews*, (**4**), CD000545.

17 Candy, S., Wright, J., Gerber, M., *et al.* (1995) A controlled double blind study of azathioprine in the management of Crohn's disease. *Gut*, **37**(5), 674–678.

18 Markowitz, J., Grancher, K., Kohn, N., *et al.* (2000) A multicenter trial of 6-mercaptopurine and prednisone in children with newly diagnosed Crohn's disease. *Gastroenterology*, **119**(4), 895–902.

19 Lemann, M., Mary, J.Y., Colombel, J.F., *et al.* (2005) A randomized, double-blind, controlled withdrawal trial in Crohn's disease patients in long-term remission on azathioprine. *Gastroenterology*, **128**(7), 1812–1818.

20 Vilien, M., Dahlerup, J.F., Munck, L.K., *et al.* (2004) Randomized controlled azathioprine withdrawal after more than two years treatment in Crohn's disease: increased relapse rate the following year. *Alimentary Pharmacology & Therapeutics*, **19**(11), 1147–1152.

21 Treton, X., Bouhnik, Y., Mary, J.Y., *et al.* (2009) Azathioprine withdrawal in patients with Crohn's disease maintained on prolonged remission: a high risk of relapse. *Clinical Gastroenterology and Hepatology*, **7**(1), 80–85.

22 Panes, J., Lopez-Sanroman, A., Bermejo, F., *et al.* (2013) Early azathioprine therapy is no more effective than placebo for newly diagnosed Crohn's disease. *Gastroenterology*, **145**(4), 766–774.e1.

23 Cosnes, J., Bourrier, A., Laharie, D., *et al.* (2013) Early administration of azathioprine vs conventional management of Crohn's disease: a randomized controlled trial. *Gastroenterology*, **145**(4), 758–765.e2.

24 Lecomte, T., Contou, J.F., Beaugerie, L., *et al.* (2003) Predictive factors of response of perianal Crohn's disease to azathioprine or 6-mercaptopurine. *Diseases of the Colon and Rectum*, **46**(11), 1469–1475.

25 Haber, C.J., Meltzer, S.J., Present, D.H., and Korelitz, B.I. (1986) Nature and course of pancreatitis caused by 6-mercaptopurine in the treatment of inflammatory bowel disease. *Gastroenterology*, **91**(4), 982–986.

26 Ledder, O.D., Lemberg, D.A., Ooi, C.Y., and Day, A.S. (2013) Are thiopurines always contraindicated after thiopurine induced pancreatitis in inflammatory bowel disease? *Journal of Pediatric Gastroenterology and Nutrition*, **57**(5), 583–586.

27 Colombel, J.F., Ferrari, N., Debuysere, H., *et al.* (2000) Genotypic analysis of thiopurine *S*-methyltransferase in patients with Crohn's disease and severe myelosuppression during azathioprine therapy. *Gastroenterology*, **118**(6), 1025–1030.

28 Leung, Y., Sparrow, M.P., Schwartz, M., and Hanauer, S.B. (2009) Long term efficacy and safety of allopurinol and azathioprine or 6-mercaptopurine in patients with inflammatory bowel disease. *Journal of Crohn's & Colitis*, **3**(3), 162–167.

29 Sparrow, M.P., Hande, S.A., Friedman, S., *et al.* (2007) Effect of allopurinol on

clinical outcomes in inflammatory bowel disease nonresponders to azathioprine or 6-mercaptopurine. *Clinical Gastroenterology and Hepatology*, **5**(2), 209–214.

30 Toruner, M., Loftus, E.V., Jr., Harmsen, W.S., *et al.* (2008) Risk factors for opportunistic infections in patients with inflammatory bowel disease. *Gastroenterology*, **134**(4), 929–936.

31 Khan, N., Abbas, A.M., Lichtenstein, G.R., *et al.* (2013) Risk of lymphoma in patients with ulcerative colitis treated with thiopurines: a nationwide retrospective cohort study. *Gastroenterology*, **145**(5), 1007–1015.e3.

32 Beaugerie, L., Brousse, N., Bouvier, A.M., *et al.* (2009) Lymphoproliferative disorders in patients receiving thiopurines for inflammatory bowel disease: a prospective observational cohort study. *Lancet*, **374**(9701), 1617–1625.

33 Kotlyar, D.S., Osterman, M.T., Diamond, R.H., *et al.* (2011) A systematic review of factors that contribute to hepatosplenic T-cell lymphoma in patients with inflammatory bowel disease. *Clinical Gastroenterology and Hepatology*, **9**(1), 36–41.e1.

34 Peyrin-Biroulet, L., Khosrotehrani, K., Carrat, F., *et al.* (2011) Increased risk for nonmelanoma skin cancers in patients who receive thiopurines for inflammatory bowel disease. *Gastroenterology*, **141**(5), 1621–1628.e5.

35 Long, M.D., Martin, C.F., Pipkin, C.A., *et al.* (2012) Risk of melanoma and nonmelanoma skin cancer among patients with inflammatory bowel disease. *Gastroenterology*, **143**(2), 390–399.e1.

36 Fraser, A.G., Orchard, T.R., Robinson, E.M., and Jewell, D.P. (2002) Long-term risk of malignancy after treatment of inflammatory bowel disease with azathioprine. *Alimentary Pharmacology & Therapeutics*, **16**(7), 1225–1232.

37 Oren, R., Arber, N., Odes, S., *et al.* (1996) Methotrexate in chronic active ulcerative colitis: a double-blind, randomized, Israeli multicenter trial. *Gastroenterology*, **110**(5), 1416–1421.

38 Manosa, M., Garcia, V., Castro, L., *et al.* (2011) Methotrexate in ulcerative colitis: a Spanish multicentric study on clinical use and efficacy. *Journal of Crohn's & Colitis*, **5**(5), 397–401.

39 Feagan, B.G., Rochon, J., Fedorak, R.N., *et al.* (1995) Methotrexate for the treatment of Crohn's disease. The North American Crohn's Study Group Investigators. *New England Journal of Medicine*, **332**(5), 292–297.

40 Feagan, B.G., Fedorak, R.N., Irvine, E.J., *et al.* (2000) A comparison of methotrexate with placebo for the maintenance of remission in Crohn's disease. The North American Crohn's Study Group Investigators. *New England Journal of Medicine*, **342**(22), 1627–1632.

41 Feagan, B.G., McDonald, J.W., Panaccione, R., *et al.* (2014) Methotrexate in combination with infliximab is no more effective than infliximab alone in patients with Crohn's disease. *Gastroenterology*, **146**(3), 681–688.e1.

42 Weiss, B., Lerner, A., Shapiro, R., *et al.* (2009) Methotrexate treatment in pediatric Crohn disease patients intolerant or resistant to purine analogues. *Journal of Pediatric Gastroenterology and Nutrition*, **48**(5), 526–530.

43 Turner, D., Grossman, A.B., Rosh, J., *et al.* (2007) Methotrexate following unsuccessful thiopurine therapy in pediatric Crohn's disease. *American Journal of Gastroenterology*, **102**(12), 2804–2812; quiz, 2803, 2813.

44 Aithal, G.P. (2011) Hepatotoxicity related to antirheumatic drugs. *Nature Reviews Rheumatology*, **7**(3), 139–150.

45 Davila-Fajardo, C.L., Swen, J.J., Cabeza Barrera, J., and Guchelaar, H.J. (2013) Genetic risk factors for drug-induced liver

injury in rheumatoid arthritis patients using low-dose methotrexate. *Pharmacogenomics*, **14**(1), 63–73.

46  Cohen, R.D., Stein, R., and Hanauer, S.B. (1999) Intravenous cyclosporin in ulcerative colitis: a five-year experience. *American Journal of Gastroenterology*, **94**(6), 1587–1592.

47  Lichtiger, S., Present, D.H., Kornbluth, A., *et al.* (1994) Cyclosporine in severe ulcerative colitis refractory to steroid therapy. *New England Journal of Medicine*, **330**(26), 1841–1845.

48  Carbonnel, F., Boruchowicz, A., Duclos, B., *et al.* (1996) Intravenous cyclosporine in attacks of ulcerative colitis: short-term and long-term responses. *Digestive Diseases and Sciences*, **41**(12), 2471–2476.

49  Arts, J., D'Haens, G., Zeegers, M., *et al.* (2004) Long-term outcome of treatment with intravenous cyclosporin in patients with severe ulcerative colitis. *Inflammatory Bowel Diseases*, **10**(2), 73–78.

50  Van Assche, G., D'Haens, G., Noman, M., *et al.* (2003) Randomized, double-blind comparison of 4 mg/kg versus 2 mg/kg intravenous cyclosporine in severe ulcerative colitis. *Gastroenterology*, **125**(4), 1025–1031.

51  D'Haens, G., Lemmens, L., Geboes, K., *et al.* (2001) Intravenous cyclosporine versus intravenous corticosteroids as single therapy for severe attacks of ulcerative colitis. *Gastroenterology*, **120**(6), 1323–1329.

52  Laharie, D., Bourreille, A., Branche, J., *et al.* (2012) Ciclosporin versus infliximab in patients with severe ulcerative colitis refractory to intravenous steroids: a parallel, open-label randomised controlled trial. *Lancet*, **380**(9857), 1909–1915.

53  Ogata, H., Kato, J., Hirai, F., *et al.* (2012) Double-blind, placebo-controlled trial of oral tacrolimus (FK506) in the management of hospitalized patients with steroid-refractory ulcerative colitis. *Inflammatory Bowel Diseases*, **18**(5), 803–808.

54  Brynskov, J., Freund, L., Rasmussen, S.N., *et al.* (1989) A placebo-controlled, double-blind, randomized trial of cyclosporine therapy in active chronic Crohn's disease. *New England Journal of Medicine*, **321**(13), 845–850.

55  Feagan, B.G., McDonald, J.W., Rochon, J., *et al.* (1994) Low-dose cyclosporine for the treatment of Crohn's disease. The Canadian Crohn's Relapse Prevention Trial Investigators. *New England Journal of Medicine*, **330**(26), 1846–1851.

56  Santos, J.V., Baudet, J.A., Casellas, F.J., *et al.* (1995) Intravenous cyclosporine for steroid-refractory attacks of Crohn's disease. Short- and long-term results. *Journal of Clinical Gastroenterology*, **20**(3), 207–210.

57  Mahdi, G., Israel, D.M., and Hassall, E. (1996) Cyclosporine and 6-mercaptopurine for active, refractory Crohn's colitis in children. *American Journal of Gastroenterology*, **91**(7), 1355–1359.

58  Lowry, P.W., Weaver, A.L., Tremaine, W.J., and Sandborn, W.J. (1999) Combination therapy with oral tacrolimus (FK506) and azathioprine or 6-mercaptopurine for treatment-refractory Crohn's disease perianal fistulae. *Inflammatory Bowel Diseases*, **5**(4), 239–245.

59  Sandborn, W.J., Present, D.H., Isaacs, K.L., *et al.* (2003) Tacrolimus for the treatment of fistulas in patients with Crohn's disease: a randomized, placebo-controlled trial. *Gastroenterology*, **125**(2), 380–388.

## Answers to Questions

1   Answer: **B**. As many as 5% of patients with thiopurine therapy may develop pancreatitis. Paradoxical worsening of colitis may be seen with aminosalicylate therapy but has not been reported with use of azathioprine or 6-mercaptopurine. Fever, arthralgia, and systemic flu-like symptoms have been reported within 1 month of initiation of thiopurine therapy. Thiopurines are also associated with a 2–4-fold increase in risk of lymphoma, primarily non-Hodgkin's lymphoma.

2   Answer: **C**. Approximately 15% of the patient population initiating thiopurines may be "shunters" who preferentially metabolize azathioprine or 6-MP towards 6-MMPN production. Such patients have subtherapeutic levels of 6-TGN and elevated levels of 6-MMPN, and dose increases of thiopurines may result in a disproportionately greater increase in 6-MMPN without significantly restoring the 6-TGN towards the therapeutic range. In such patients, addition of allopurinol can reverse the shunting and restore therapeutic 6-TGN levels. However, initiation of allopurinol should be accompanied by a dose reduction of the original immunomodulator dose by 50–75% to avoid severe myelosuppression.

3   Answer: **C**. Even though patients with low or intermediate TPMT enzyme activity are more susceptible to myelosuppression, most patients who develop a low WBC count on thiopurine therapy have normal TPMT genotype. In addition, low WBC counts have been first seen as long as 1 year or more after initiation of thiopurine therapy. Elevated levels of 6-MMPN are associated with hepatotoxicity but not myelosuppression in patients on thiopurine therapy.

4   Answer: **B**. In a double-blind placebo-controlled trial that randomized 141 patients with active CD to methotrexate or placebo, Feagan *et al.* demonstrated that at the end of 16 weeks, 39% of patients in the methotrexate group were in clinical remission compared with 19% of patients on placebo [39]. In the maintenance phase of the trial utilizing 15 mg of intramuscular methotrexate weekly, a larger proportion of methotrexate users were in remission at 1 year compared with those receiving placebo. In the COMMIT study of patients with CD initiating prednisone treatment, a combination of methotrexate and infliximab was similar in efficacy to infliximab monotherapy [41].

8

# Biologic Therapies

---

## Clinical Take Home Messages

- Large and rigorously conducted randomized controlled trials have established the efficacy of three biologic monoclonal antibodies to tumor necrosis factor alpha (TNF-α) in inducing and maintaining remission in Crohn's disease (CD) (infliximab, adalimumab, certolizumab pegol) and three in ulcerative colitis (UC) (infliximab, adalimumab, golimumab).
- Screening for latent tuberculosis and hepatitis B infection is essential prior to starting treatment with anti-TNF biologics.
- Loss of response to anti-TNF biologics, confirmed by objective evidence of active inflammation, can be managed by optimizing therapy based on testing for the presence of antidrug antibodies and trough levels for infliximab or adalimumab. Loss of response due to immunogenicity can be managed by switching to a different anti-TNF agent while persistent inflammation in the setting of adequate trough levels of drug should prompt switching to a drug with a different mechanism of action (such as integrin inhibitors). Inadequate trough levels in the absence of antidrug antibodies can be managed by dose escalation with infliximab or adalimumab.

- Combination therapy of azathioprine and infliximab in immunomodulator-naive patients with CD is associated with higher rates of corticosteroid-free remission and mucosal healing compared with either agent given alone.
- Natalizumab, an $\alpha_4$-integrin inhibitor, is efficacious in the induction and maintenance of response in CD but is associated with a risk of rare but usually fatal progressive multifocal leukoencephalopathy (PML), particularly in those who are seropositive for the JC virus or have prior exposure to immunosuppressive therapy.
- Vedolizumab, a selective $\alpha_4\beta_7$-integrin inhibitor, is effective in the induction and maintenance of remission in both CD and UC. Owing to gut-selective integrin inhibition, it may not be associated with risk of PML.

---

The availability of biologic therapies has revolutionized the management of inflammatory bowel disease (IBD), improving our ability to achieve remission and mucosal healing and reducing the need for IBD-related surgeries and hospitalizations in both

Crohn's disease (CD) and ulcerative colitis (UC). Large and rigorously conducted randomized controlled trials (RCTs) have established the efficacy of three biologic monoclonal antibodies to tumor necrosis factor alpha (TNF-α) in inducing and maintaining remission in CD (infliximab, adalimumab, certolizumab pegol) and three in UC (infliximab, adalimumab, golimumab). There have been few head-to-head comparisons of biologic therapies with conventional immunosuppressive agents and there are only limited data examining comparative effectiveness within the different biologic therapies. The biologics vary in their induction regimen, maintenance dosing, and available dose escalation to loss of response (Table 8.1).

## Infliximab

Infliximab is a chimeric mouse/human monoclonal IgG1 antibody against TNF-α, comprising a 25% variable murine Fab fragment linked to 75% human Fc fragment [1]. It exerts its action by binding to both membrane-bound and free TNF-α, preventing it from binding to its two receptors – TNFR1 and TNFR2. The Fc regions present in infliximab and adalimumab also mediate apoptosis in cells expressing TNF-α; this effect is not seen with certolizumab pegol, which lacks the Fc fragment. All three agents reduce levels of TNF-α, an important mediator of inflammation in IBD. Anti-TNF drugs reduce levels of interleukin (IL)-6, other acute-phase reactants such as C-reactive protein (CRP), and inhibit production of IL-1β in response to lipopolysaccharide stimulation [1]. Infliximab treatment also reduces the expression of stress proteins in response to injury such as the neutrophil–gelatinase-associated lipocalin [2].

Infliximab is administered intravenously at a starting dose of 5 mg kg$^{-1}$. Lower doses, although used in rheumatoid arthritis, have not been shown to be effective in IBD. The loading dose is administered at weeks 0, 2, and 6. Initially used as an episodic maintenance strategy with on-demand administration, it was soon realized that this was associated with a high rate of immunogenicity, infusion reactions, and loss of efficacy. Consequently, the practice of regular maintenance dosing was adopted where it is administered intravenously every 8 weeks. The dose of infliximab can be escalated by either increasing the dose administered at each infusion up to 10 mg kg$^{-1}$ or shortening the interval between the infusions to as frequent as every 4 weeks. Both strategies have similar efficacy [3]. Compliance with therapy is essential as irregular exposure to medication is associated with reduced durability of treatment [4]. Premedication with corticosteroids and concomitant immunomodulator therapy reduce rates of formation of antibodies to infliximab (ATI) [previously termed human anti-chimeric antibodies (HACAs)] and may preserved durability of therapy [5].

### Efficacy in Ulcerative Colitis

The pivotal ACT 1 and ACT 2 trials established the efficacy of infliximab in UC. In each trial, 364 patients with moderate to severe active UC were randomly assigned to receive placebo or 5 or 10 mg kg$^{-1}$ of infliximab, administered every 8 weeks after the standard induction doses. The trial duration was 30 weeks for ACT 2 and 54 weeks for ACT 1. In the ACT 1 trial, at week 8, the primary endpoint of clinical response was met in 69% and 62% of patients in the group receiving 5 and 10 mg kg$^{-1}$ of infliximab, respectively, compared with 37% in patients receiving placebo. Similar results were observed in the ACT2 trial [6] (Figure 8.1). There was no difference in infections or other adverse effects between the two groups. The cumulative incidence of colectomy

Table 8.1 Dose and route of administration of biologic agents in Crohn's disease and ulcerative colitis.

| Agent | Mechanism of action | Route of administration | Induction dosing | Maintenance dosing | Management of loss of response |
|---|---|---|---|---|---|
| Infliximab | Antibody to TNF-$\alpha$ | IV | 5 mg kg$^{-1}$ at weeks 0, 2, and 6 | 5 mg kg$^{-1}$ every 8 weeks | Dose increase up to 10 mg kg$^{-1}$, interval shortening up to 4 weeks |
| Adalimumab | Antibody to TNF-$\alpha$ | SC | 160 mg at week 0, 80 mg at week 2 | 40 mg every 2 weeks | Dose increase to 40 mg weekly |
| Certolizumab pegol[a] | Antibody to TNF-$\alpha$ | SC | 400 mg at weeks 0 and 2 | 400 mg every 4 weeks | 400 mg booster at week 2 |
| Golimumab[b] | Antibody to TNF-$\alpha$ | SC | 200 mg at week 0, 100 mg at week 2 | 100 mg at week 6, then 100 mg every 4 weeks | – |
| Natalizumab[a] | Anti-integrin ($\alpha_4$-integrin) | IV | 300 mg at weeks 0 and 4 | 300 mg every 4 weeks | – |
| Vedolizumab | Anti-integrin ($\alpha_4\beta_7$-integrin) | IV | 300 mg at weeks 0, 2, and 6 | 300 mg every 8 weeks | – |

[a] Crohn's disease only.
[b] Ulcerative colitis only.

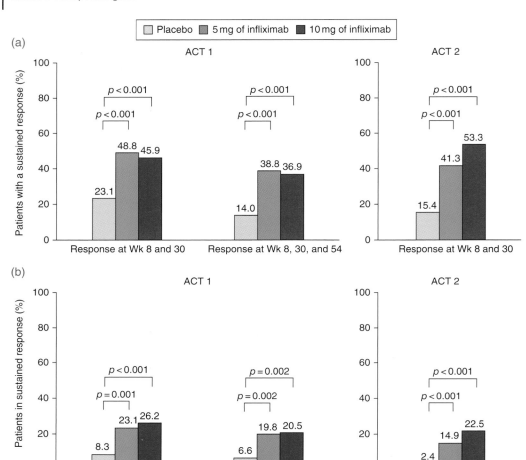

**Figure 8.1** Efficacy of infliximab maintenance in ulcerative colitis: proportion of patients with a sustained clinical response (a) and in sustained clinical remission (b) in ACT 1 and ACT 2. *Source:* Rutgeerts *et al.* 2005 [6]. Reproduced with permission of Massachusetts Medical Society.

was also lower in the infliximab-treated group (10%) compared with placebo (17%) [7]. Not only was infliximab associated with clinical response, but also higher rates of mucosal healing and early mucosal healing at week 8 were associated with decreased need for colectomy through week 54 [8]. Similar efficacy has been established in pediatric UC with a similar dose and frequency of administration [9].

Most studies have evaluated infliximab in outpatients with moderate to severe disease, but a few RCTs have examined its efficacy in the treatment of acute severe steroid-refractory UC in hospitalized patients. In a pilot trial of 11 patients, half of the patients who received infliximab achieved treatment success at 2 weeks compared with none of the patients who received placebo [10]. A larger RCT by Jarnerot *et al.* demonstrated a lower 3-month colectomy rate among patients treated with a single dose of infliximab 5 mg kg$^{-1}$ (29%) compared with placebo (67%) [11]. Long-term follow-up revealed continued benefit through 3 years, although a majority of the treatment benefit was short term [12].

**Efficacy in Crohn's Disease**

A wealth of data supports the use of infliximab in luminal and fistulizing CD. van Dullemen *et al.*, recognizing the elevated circulating concentrations of TNF-α in patients with CD, reported the first use of a chimeric monoclonal antibody directed against TNF-α (cA2) in 10 patients with CD [13]. Normalization of the CD activity index (CDAI) and healing of ulcerations were observed in eight patients within 4 weeks of a single dose. Targan *et al.* reported the first randomized trial of 108 patients with moderate to severe CD who received infliximab at 5, 10, or 20 mg kg$^{-1}$, or placebo. At 4 weeks, 81% of patients in the 5 mg kg$^{-1}$ arm had a clinical response compared with 17% on placebo, a remarkable benefit given the modest efficacy of prior therapies in CD [14]. However, a large proportion of patients who received a single infusion of infliximab relapsed at a mean of 8.5 weeks after the infusion. The landmark ACCENT I trial then demonstrated efficacy of infliximab maintenance therapy. A total of 573 patients with moderate to severe CD were treated with an infusion of infliximab 5 mg kg$^{-1}$. Patients responding to the infusion at week 2 were randomized to receive infliximab 5 mg kg$^{-1}$ or placebo at weeks 2 and 6, followed by the options of infliximab 5 or 10 mg kg$^{-1}$ or placebo for maintenance therapy every 8 weeks until week 46. A total of 58% of patients responded to the initial infusion of infliximab. At week 30, 21% of patients in the placebo arm were in remission compared with 39% and 45% of those in the 5 and 10 mg kg$^{-1}$ maintenance arms [15]

(Figure 8.2). Subsequent analysis confirmed that regular maintenance infliximab was associated with improved quality of life and a higher rate of complete mucosal healing at week 54, along with a trend towards reduced rates of hospitalization [16]. Episodic infliximab infusions were associated with a greater incidence of antibody formation [17], reduced long-term efficacy, and an increased risk of infusion reactions [18].

Several observational cohorts have confirmed the durable efficacy of infliximab in maintaining remission in luminal CD. In a long-term study of 614 patients treated with infliximab, sustained benefit was observed in 63% of those receiving long-term treatment. Continued infliximab use was associated with higher rates of steroid discontinuation and a decreased need for hospitalizations and surgery [19]. The annual risk for loss of infliximab response was 13% [20]. Among those losing response, 76% were able to regain response after dose intensification [21, 22], with many able to maintain their response for 1 year or longer [23]. Therapeutic drug monitoring has proven to be a successful strategy to assess mechanisms of loss of response and to optimize infliximab dosing (Figure 8.3). Lower trough drug concentrations of infliximab are associated with lower rates of response and endoscopic healing. Reduced drug concentrations may be seen in the setting of immunogenicity and formation of antibodies to infliximab. In a large series of 1487 trough serum samples from 483 patients with CD, three-quarters (77%) had a detectable trough concentration whereas 23% had an undetectable infliximab level [24]. Over two-thirds of those with an undetectable trough level showed the presence of anti-infliximab antibodies. Therapeutic trough concentrations of 3 μg ml$^{-1}$ or higher were associated with higher rates of remission. Patients who had low trough levels due to antibodies benefit from a switch to a different anti-TNF agent, as these antibodies are usually not cross-reactive across the

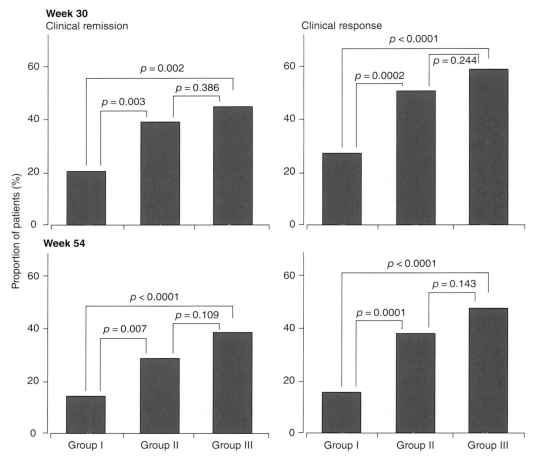

**Figure 8.2** Efficacy of infliximab in Crohn's disease: clinical response and clinical remission for week-2 responders in the ACCENT I randomized trial. Groups I, II, and III indicate patients randomized to placebo, 5 mg kg$^{-1}$, and 10 mg kg$^{-1}$ maintenance regimens, respectively. *Source:* Adapted from Hanauer *et al.* 2002 [15]. Reproduced with permission of Elsevier.

different anti-TNF biologic agents. Patients who have low trough levels due to non-immune-mediated clearance such as fecal loss in severe disease may benefit from dose escalation whereas patients who have persistent inflammation in the setting of a therapeutic trough drug level of 3 μg ml$^{-1}$ or higher are unlikely to respond to another anti-TNF biologic and merit addition or a switch to an agent belonging to a different therapeutic class [25].

Limited comparative effectiveness data exist to guide the different therapeutic choices either within the different anti-TNF agents or between such biologics and immunomodulators. The SONIC trial was the first such head-to-head comparison of infliximab with conventional therapy randomizing patients with CD naive to immunomodulator therapy to azathioprine, infliximab, or a combination of both agents [22]. At the end of the study, 57% of patients

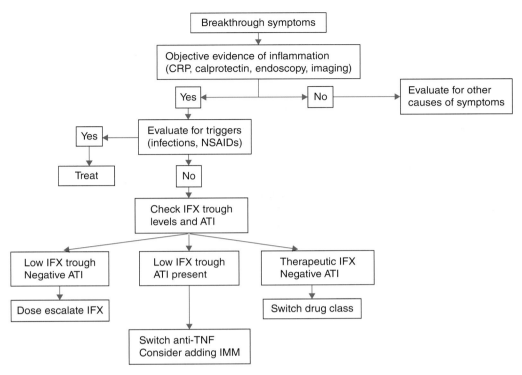

**Figure 8.3** Algorithm for management of loss of response to infliximab. CRP, C-reactive protein; NSAIDs, non-steroidal anti-inflammatory drugs; IFX, infliximab; ATI, antibodies to inlfiximab; anti-TNF, monoclonal antibodies to TNF-α; IMM, immunomodulator.

receiving combination therapy achieved the primary study outcome of steroid-free clinical remission compared with 44% receiving infliximab alone and 30% of those receiving azathioprine alone (Figure 8.4). Similar trends were observed at week 50. Mucosal healing was more frequent in the combination therapy and infliximab arms compared with those receiving azathioprine. This landmark study also established that combination immunomodulator–infliximab therapy was associated with reduced rates of antibodies to infliximab and higher trough levels. The benefit of concomitant immunomodulator use along with infliximab was supported by trials examining the impact of withdrawal of concomitant immunosuppression on infliximab maintenance. Although a similar proportion of patients

were able to remain on infliximab at 2 years without needing a change in dosing interval in an open-label randomized trial, infliximab trough levels were higher and the CRP level was lower in the group that continued combination maintenance treatment than in those who were continued only on monotherapy [26]. Infliximab also appears to be effective in pediatric CD disease, with higher rates of response at weeks 10 and 54 compared with that seen in the adult infliximab trials [27].

The efficacy of infliximab in fistulizing CD was established in the ACCENT II study, in which continued infliximab maintenance at 5 mg kg$^{-1}$ every 8 weeks was associated with a higher rate of absence of draining fistulas (36%) than with placebo administration (19%) [28]. Infliximab was efficacious in

(a)

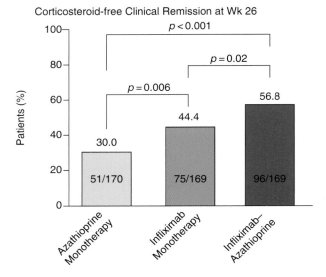

(b)

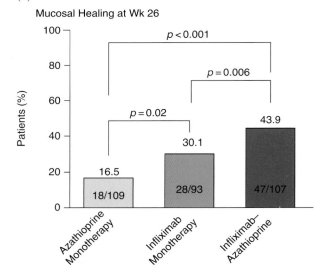

Figure 8.4 Comparative effectiveness of infliximab, azathioprine, and combination therapy: corticosteroid-free clinical remission (a) and mucosal healing (b) at week 26 in the SONIC trial. *Source:* Colombel *et al.* 2010 [63]. Reproduced with permission of Massachusetts Medical Society.

achieving short-term closure of recto-vaginal fistulas [29]. In a long-term observational cohort of 156 patients receiving infliximab for perianal fistulizing CD, after a median follow-up of 250 weeks, 69% had closure of at least one fistula. The probability of fistula closure at 1 and 5 years was 40% and 65%, respectively [30].

**Safety**

Adverse events with biologic use are uncommon but may be serious. Infusion reactions occur in 5–20% of patients treated with infliximab and may occur either during the infusion or in the days following [31, 32]. Acute infusion reactions usually occur during or shortly after an infusion and manifest as chest tightness or pain, shortness of breath, flushing, urticaria, and fever. Delayed infusion reactions have similar symptoms, but may include arthralgia and serum sickness-like features, and occur 2–14 days after infusion. Anaphylactic reactions are rare [31]. Infusion reactions are more frequent in the presence of antibodies to infliximab but do not require the presence of neutralizing antibodies. Episodic therapy increases the risk of infusion reactions whereas concomitant immunosuppressive therapy or pretreatment with hydrocortisone may reduce antibody formation and the risk of infusion reactions. Acute infusion reactions usually respond to hydrocortisone, acetaminophen, and diphenhydramine. As the antibodies to infliximab are typically not cross-reactive with other anti-TNF biologics, recurrence of infusion reaction-like symptoms with the other injectable anti-TNF agents is unlikely.

Infections are another important adverse effect of biologics; the risk is modestly further increased with addition of immunomodulators in UC but not CD, and with concomitant corticosteroid therapy in both diseases [33]. A multi-institutional collaboration assessing patients receiving these agents as treatment for a variety of autoimmune diseases suggested the absolute risk of hospitalization for serious infection to be 11 per 100 person-years for new users of anti-TNF agents in IBD compared with 10 per 100 person-years for comparators that included other immunosuppressives [34]. In a large cohort of 500 patients initiated on infliximab therapy, 48 developed infections; the most common serious infections were pneumonia, viral infections, abdominal abscesses, and sepsis [32]. In the most recent analysis of the Crohn's Therapy, Resource, Evaluation, and Assessment Tool (TREAT) registry, a prospective observational cohort of patients in the United States, among 3420 patients initiating infliximab and totaling 17 712 patient-years of follow-up, infliximab use was associated with a modest increase in risk of infection [hazard ration (HR) 1.43, 95% confidence interval (CI) 1.11–1.84] with an absolute risk of two infections per 100 person-years of exposure. The most common infections were pneumonia (19%), abdominal abscesses (9%), and sepsis (7%). Serious mycobacterial or fungal infections were uncommon but included tuberculosis and atypical mycobacteria, in addition to *Pneumocystis jiroveci* infection, systemic candidiasis, and other fungemia [35]. In particular, reactivation of tuberculosis may occur with biologic therapy. Consequently, all patients must be screened for latent tuberculosis prior to initiation using either the tuberculin skin test or an interferon-gamma release assay (QuantiFERON-TB Gold, T-SPOT), with the latter assays being less prone to influence by immunosuppression. Individuals testing positive for latent tuberculosis should receive treatment with isoniazid or rifampin prior to beginning anti-TNF therapy. A meta-analysis of opportunistic infections in patients enrolled in clinical trials of biologic anti-TNF therapy revealed a twofold increase in rate of opportunistic infections, but the number needed to harm was high at 500 [36]. Hepatitis B reactivation has also been seen in patients who are carriers and initiate anti-TNF therapy. Screening for carrier state or past infection is important prior to the start of biologic therapy. Current or past hepatitis C infection is not affected by biologic use.

Treatment-related malignancy in association with long-term therapy is another important concern with biologic agents. However, data obtained so far have been reassuring with respect to most cancers. In a Danish cohort of 651 patients treated with infliximab, four developed cancer compared with 5.9 expected [standardized incidence ratio (SIR) 0.7, 95% CI 0.2–1.7]. Pooled analysis of clinical trials and other observational cohorts does not suggest an overall increase in risk of solid organ tumors with infliximab [33, 37]. Infliximab use is associated with a modest increase in the risk of non-Hodgkin's lymphoma (SIR 3.23, 95% CI 1.5–6.9), but the absolute risk remains low (6.1 per 10 000 patient-years). Anti-TNF biologic use is also associated with a twofold increase in the risk of melanoma [38].

Anti-TNF biologics can be associated with paradoxical immune-mediated side effects, which include a drug-induced lupus-like reaction and psoriasis. The mechanism behind the emergence of these autoimmune diseases is unclear, particularly since biologics are effective in the management of some of these same diseases. A new-onset skin rash, particularly palmo-plantar in distribution, in patients on anti-TNF biologic therapy should prompt consideration of anti-TNF-induced psoriasis. This may respond to topical treatment, although in a significant minority of patients cessation of the offending agent may be required and the lesions may recur with a different anti-TNF biologic. Drug-induced lupus erythematosus (DILE) related to anti-TNF biologics is less frequently associated positively with anti-histone antibody (when compared with other DILE), but patients frequently demonstrate an elevated antinuclear antibody and anti-double-stranded DNA antibody. Often, this paradoxical complication requires cessation of the offending agent. Subsequent rechallenge with another anti-TNF biologic may result in recurrence in a small subset of patients, and changing therapy to a different pharmacologic class may be preferable. In an RCT, infliximab was associated with worse outcomes in patients with moderate to severe congestive heart failure; hence decompensated heart disease is a contraindication for the use of these therapies [39]. Demyelinating disease and active cancer are also contraindications for their use.

## Adalimumab

Adalimumab is a humanized monoclonal IgG1 antibody against TNF-α. It is administered subcutaneously with a loading dose in adults of 160 mg at week 0 and 80 mg at week 2, followed by a maintenance regimen of a 40 mg subcutaneous injection every 2 weeks beginning from week 4. This dosing is distinct from adalimumab use for other autoimmune diseases where the loading dose is usually not administered. In CD, the response rate is inferior without the administration of a loading dose. Similarly to that observed with infliximab, the annual risk of loss of response to adalimumab is 20% per patient-year. Loss of response can be treated by dose intensification to 40 mg weekly, allowing for regaining of response in three-quarters of patients [40]. Adverse reactions to adalimumab are similar to those to infliximab. Reactions specific to adalimumab include injection site reactions, which occur in 20% of patients. Similar to infliximab, therapeutic drug monitoring may play a role in optimizing treatment strategy and guiding dose escalation, although less is known about the optimal drug level and management of antidrug antibodies.

### Efficacy in Ulcerative Colitis

The efficacy of adalimumab in UC was first established in small open-label series of patients losing response to infliximab [25, 41, 42]. Subsequently, an RCT by Reinisch *et al.* randomized 186 patients with moderate to severe UC and a Mayo score of ≥6 to adalimumab or placebo. At week 8, 19% of patients in the adalimumab arm compared with 9% treated with placebo were in remission [43]. The rates of remission were higher in anti-TNF-naive patients than in those with prior anti-TNF failure. In the ULTRA 2 study of maintenance adalimumab, 22% of patients in the adalimumab 40 mg sucutaneously every other week arm were in clinical remission at week 52 compared with 12% of patients treated with placebo.

### Efficacy in Crohn's Disease

Multiple clinical trials have examined the efficacy of adalimumab in luminal and fistulizing CD. The CLASSIC 1 trial randomized 299 patients with moderate to severe CD naive to anti-TNF therapy to three different regimens of adalimumab given as subcutaneous injections, (40 mg/20 mg, 80 mg/40 mg, and 160 mg/80 mg, or placebo). At week 4, the primary endpoint of remission was met in 18% of patients in the 40 mg/20 mg arm, 24% in the 80 mg/40 mg arm, and 36% in the 160 mg/80 mg arm compared with 12% of patients receiving placebo [44]. The only treatment arm that met statistical significance was the 160 mg/80 mg loading dose, establishing this as the standard induction regimen. The GAIN trial examined the efficacy of adalimumab induction in 325 patients with failure or intolerance to infliximab therapy. At 4 weeks, 21% of patients in the adalimumab group versus 7% of patients in the placebo group achieved remission, yielding an absolute difference of 14%. The smaller magnitude of benefit in the GAIN trial compared with the CLASSIC trial highlighted the reduced rate of response with subsequent anti-TNF use in patients who had already experienced treatment failure with an anti-TNF agent. Furthermore, the rate of response to adalimumab in patients with primary non-response to infliximab in the GAIN trial was lower than that in patients who stopped infliximab for other reasons or had secondary loss of response [45].

The maintenance regimen of adalimumab was established in the CLASSIC II and CHARM trials. In the CLASSIC II trial, 55 patients from the CLASSIC I trial who were in remission at week 4 were re-randomized to adalimumab 40 mg every other week, 40 mg weekly, or placebo and followed through to 56 weeks. Patients who were not in remission

at the end of CLASSIC I were allowed openlabel adalimumab 40 mg every other week with the dose increased to 40 mg every week for loss of response. At the end of the study, among the 55 randomized patients, 79% in the adalimumab every other week arm and 83% of those in the weekly adalimumab arm were in remission at week 56 compared with 44% of those treated with placebo. The CHARM trial included open-label 80 mg at week 0 and 40 mg at week 2 as the induction regimen for all patients and randomized patients to then receive 40 mg every other week, 40 mg weekly or placebo therapy through week 56. A larger proportion of patients in the 40 mg every other week arm (36%) and 40 mg every week arm (41%) were in remission at week 56 compared with placebo (12%) [46] (Figure 8.5). Similarly to the results observed with infliximab therapy, continued maintenance was more effective than initial induction followed by reintroduction in the setting of loss of response [47]. Further analyses of CHARM data found that adalimumab was effective in improving health-related quality of life and reducing the need for hospitalization and surgery.

Open-label observational cohorts confirmed the efficacy of adalimumab in clinical practice, and demonstrated that even if dose adjustment is required in up to one-third of the patients at the end of 1 year, a significant proportion are able to regain and maintain response. With increasing recognition of mucosal healing as an important outcome, the EXTEND trial randomized 135 patients with moderate to severe ileocolonic CD to treatment with adalimumab 40 mg every other week or placebo after the standard induction regimen. At week 12, mucosal healing was observed in 27% of patients receiving adalimumab compared with 13% given placebo; this difference remained striking at week 52, with endoscopic remission rates of 24% and 0%, respectively. In addition to demonstrating the efficacy of adalimumab in achieving mucosal healing, this trial is also significant in

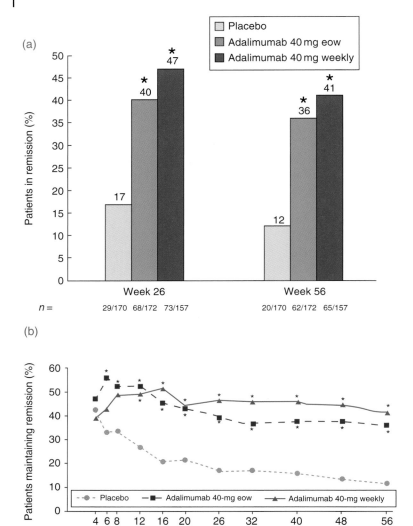

**Figure 8.5** Efficacy of adalimumab maintenance therapy in Crohn's disease. Clinical remission at weeks 26 and 56 (a) and clinical remission over time (b) in randomized responder population (week 4 responders) in the CHARM trial. *Source:* Adapted from Colombel *et al.* 2007 [46]. Reproduced with permission of Elsevier.

that it is one of the first in which mucosal healing in CD was the primary endpoint.

Adalimumab also has demonstrated efficacy in fistulizing CD, although the data are less rigorous than those for infliximab [48]. The IMAgINE 1 study evaluated adalimumab in pediatric CD and demonstrated efficacy similar to that observed in the adult population [49].

## Certolizumab Pegol

Certolizumab pegol is a pegylated Fab fragment of a monoclonal antibody to TNF-α. Owing to lack of an Fc fragment, certolizumab pegol does not activate, complement, or mediate antibody-dependent cellular cytotoxicity and apoptosis, in contrast to infliximab and adalimumab. It is administered subcutaneously with an induction dose of 400 mg at weeks 0 and 2 followed by 400 mg every 4 weeks for maintenance. Adverse effects with certolizumab pegol are similar to those associated with adalimumab and infliximab. Although multiple clinical trials have examined the efficacy of certolizumab pegol in CD, there are only limited data supporting its use in UC.

### Efficacy in Crohn's Disease

Drawing from the experience of a previous trial in which certolizumab pegol was effective in the subgroup of patients with elevated baseline CRP, the PRECISE 1 study randomized 662 adults with moderate to severe CD to receive certolizumab pegol 400 mg at weeks 0, 2, and 4 followed by treatment every 4 weeks. Among patients with a baseline CRP level of at least 10 mg l$^{-1}$, 37% of patients in the certolizumab pegol group had a response at week 6 compared with 26% in the placebo group. The rates of response at week 26 also favored certolizumab pegol (22% and 12%, respectively), with borderline statistical significance. There was no difference in the rates of remission between the two groups at either time point [50], a finding also seen in subsequent independent trials. The PRECISE 2 study evaluated maintenance through week 26 in patients who responded to the initial dosing. Among those with elevated CRP at baseline, the rates of response at week 26 were significantly higher in the certolizumab pegol group (62%) compared with the placebo group (34%) ($p$ <0.001). This efficacy was independent of concomitant immunosuppressant use or prior exposure to infliximab. Subsequent extension of this study through 18 months revealed continued efficacy in maintaining remission [51]. The PRECISE 4 study demonstrated that in the setting of disease relapse on certolizumab pegol maintenance, efficacy could be recaptured and maintained through week 52 in 55% of patients who were reinduced with one additional dose [52]. Subgroup analysis of the PRECISE 2 trial firmly established duration of disease to be an important predictor of response to anti-TNF therapy. Maintenance of response was achieved in 89% of patients who were within the first year of diagnosis of CD but only 57% in those with disease duration of 4 years or longer.

## Golimumab

Golimumab is a humanized monoclonal antibody to anti-TNF that is useful in the treatment of rheumatoid arthritis and psoriasis. The PURSUIT clinical trial program examined its efficacy in UC. In this multicenter RCT, patients with moderate to severe UC with a Mayo score of 6–12 and an endoscopic subscore of ≥2 were randomized to placebo or one of three doses of golimumab at weeks 0 and 2, namely 100/50, 200/100, or 400/200 mg. In the phase 3 efficacy analysis comprising 771 patients, 52% and 55% in the golimumab 200/100 and 400/200 mg arms, respectively, achieved clinical response compared with 30% of those treated with placebo [53]. Patients who responded to induction therapy were able to maintain response through week 54 in significantly greater numbers if they received 50 or 100 mg of golimumab administered every 4 weeks compared with placebo [54]; the 100 mg dose arm achieved greater rates of remission and mucosal healing at week 54 [54].

## Natalizumab

$\alpha_4$-integrins are important cell adhesion molecules that mediate the migration of white blood cells across the vascular endothelium. Given the central role of this process in intestinal inflammation, antibodies to $\alpha_4$-integrins were of great interest as a target for the treatment of CD. Natalizumab was the first monoclonal antibody to $\alpha_4$-integrins that was studied for the treatment of CD. It is administered intravenously in a dose of 300 mg every 4 weeks. Although initial trials demonstrated efficacy, reports emerged of a serious neurologic complication, progressive multifocal leukoencephalopathy (PML). This is a progressive, disabling, and often fatal neurologic condition due to reactivation of latent JC virus infection. Natalizumab was withdrawn from use following these initial reports. However, after subsequent post-marketing surveillance revealed the incidence of PML to be low (1 per 1000 person-years), natalizumab was reintroduced with restrictions, including enrollment of treatment providers in a certification program. All patients who developed PML were seropositive for the JC virus; to date, there have been no cases in seronegative individuals. Routine testing for JC virus exposure allows stratification of risk in individuals when this therapy is a potential option. Those seronegative for JC virus appear to have a risk of 1:10 000 or even lower, as no PML cases have been reported in seronegative individuals. If natalizumab treatment is begun in such patients, testing for the JC virus antibody should be repeated every 6 months. In contrast, in individuals who are seropositive, the risk of PML in the setting of prior immunosuppressant use and natalizumab use for 2 years or longer is considerable, reaching 1:100–1:500 after 2 years, and long-term exposure to natalizumab should be avoided in such patients.

RCTs examining efficacy of natalizumab have been restricted to CD. Two trials published in 2003–2005 demonstrated natalizumab to be an effective treatment for induction of remission in patients with moderate to severe CD [55, 56]. In the first trial, 905 patients were randomized to receive 300 mg of natalizumab or placebo at weeks 0, 4, and 8. A 70-point reduction in the CDAI was observed in 56% of patients in the natalizumab group at week 10; however, the rate of response to placebo was also high at 49% and the trial failed to meet its primary endpoint. In the second trial, 339 patients were randomized to the same treatment regimens through week 56, and higher rates of sustained response and remission were seen at week 36. The ENCORE trial established the efficacy of natalizumab in induction of remission among patients with moderate to severe CD who had an elevated CRP at baseline. Sustained remission at week 12 was seen in 26% of patients treated with natalizumab compared with 16% of those treated with placebo.

## Vedolizumab

Vedolizumab is a gut-selective $\alpha_4\beta_7$-integrin inhibitor that does not interfere with lymphocyte trafficking in the central nervous system. Theoretically, this agent should not increase the risk of PML. The GEMINI 1 study included an induction phase with vedolizumab 300 mg given intravenously at days 1 and 15 and a maintenance phase with vedolizumab 300 mg every 4 or 8 weeks [57]. The GEMINI 2 study was a parallel trial in CD and followed a similar study design [58]. In UC, 47% of patients in the vedolizumab group achieved response compared with 26% of patients treated with placebo. At week 52, the remission rates were similar in the every 8 weeks and every 4 weeks treatment arms and both were significantly greater than with placebo, yielding an absolute difference of 26% for the every 8 weeks maintenance strategy (Figure 8.6). In CD, clinical remission at week 6 was seen in 15% of patients treated with vedolizumab compared with 7% of patients treated with placebo, suggesting a more delayed onset of action compared with UC. However, at week 52, both the every 8 weeks and every

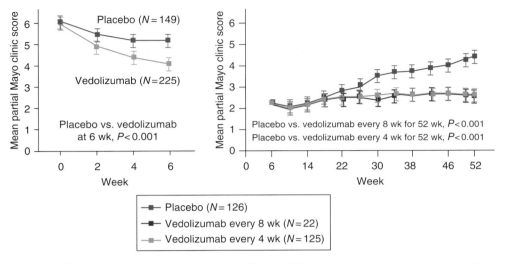

**Figure 8.6** Efficacy of vedolizumab in ulcerative colitis: the GEMINI trial demonstrating improvement in partial Mayo score with placebo and vedolizumab every 4 weeks and every 8 weeks in patients with ulcerative colitis. *Source:* Feagan *et al.* 2013 [57]. Reproduced with permission of Massachusetts Medical Society.

4 weeks vedolizumab maintenance arms were superior to placebo and met statistical significance, although the absolute difference between the groups was less than that seen in patients with UC. Within the GEMINI clinical trials, no incremental benefit in achieving clinical remission was noted with use of concomitant immunomodulator therapy. Side effects have been infrequent with vedolizumab use, with nasopharyngitis the most common infection observed.

## Newer Therapies

Other monoclonal antibodies have demonstrated significant promise in phase 2b and ongoing phase 3 trials and seem likely to become available for the treatment of CD and UC in the relatively near future. Etrolizumab is a humanized monoclonal antibody that is selective for the $\beta_7$ subunit of the integrins, allowing it to target both $\alpha_4\beta_7$ and $\alpha_E\beta_7$. In an RCT examining its efficacy in moderate to severe UC, 21% of patients in the etrolizumab 100 mg group were in

clinical remission at week 10 compared with none in the placebo group [59]. Serious adverse infections were uncommon. Larger phase 3 trials are currently under way.

Ustekinumab is a human monoclonal antibody against IL-12 and IL-23 that has demonstrated efficacy in both induction and maintenance of remission in phase 3 clinical trials for CD. A phase 2b RCT randomized 526 patients who had failed anti-TNF treatment to receive an intravenous dose of ustekinumab 1, 3, or 6 mg kg$^{-1}$ or placebo at week 0 [60]. Week 6 responders were randomized to receive 90 mg ustekinumab or placebo at weeks 8 and 16. The proportion of patients who achieved clinical response at week 6 was 40% in the ustekinumab 6 mg kg$^{-1}$ arm compared with 24% in the placebo arm. Treatment with ustekinumab through an additional 16 weeks was superior to placebo in maintaining clinical remission and response.

Tofacitinib is an oral Janus kinase (JAK) inhibitor that inhibits JAK1 and JAK3. Data from early phase 2 clinical trials suggest promising efficacy, particularly in ulcerative colitis [61], and larger phase 3 clinical trials are under way.

## Case Studies and Multiple Choice Questions

1   Which of the following adverse reactions have *not* been reported with the use of infliximab therapy in inflammatory bowel disease?
   A  Psoriasis.
   B  Lupus-like reaction.
   C  Serum sickness.
   D  Drug-induced systemic sclerosis.

2   Brenda is a 55-year-old woman with colonic Crohn's disease presenting to you for consultation. Her past history is significant for atrial fibrillation that is currently under control with metoprolol, early multiple sclerosis without significant neurologic deficit, and hepatitis C. She also has a history of breast cancer diagnosed at age 40 years treated with lumpectomy, and a history of Hodgkin's lymphoma in her father. She inquires about going on adalimumab therapy for her Crohn's disease due to persistent symptoms on thiopurine. Which of the following would represent an absolute contraindication to the use of anti-TNF therapy in her?
   A  History of atrial fibrillation.
   B  Prior breast cancer.
   C  Multiple sclerosis.

   D  Hepatitis C.
   E  Family history of lymphoma.

3   Which of the following risk factors do not increase the risk of progressive multifocal leukoencephalopathy in patients on therapy with natalizumab for Crohn's disease?
   A  Duration of therapy of at least 2 years.
   B  Prior immunosuppression.
   C  JC virus seropositivity.
   D  Prior use of vedolizumab.
   E  None of the above.

4   The following statements are true about vedolizumab except:
   A  It is effective in the induction and maintenance of remission in ulcerative colitis.
   B  Combination therapy with an immunomodulator is associated with higher rates of response and remission at 6 weeks in ulcerative colitis.
   C  It is not associated with an increased risk of progressive multifocal leukoencephalopathy.
   D  It is effective in the induction and maintenance of remission in Crohn's disease.

# References

1 Lee, T.W., and Fedorak, R.N. (2010) Tumor necrosis factor-alpha monoclonal antibodies in the treatment of inflammatory bowel disease: clinical practice pharmacology. *Gastroenterology Clinics of North America*, **39**(3), 543–557.

2 Bolignano, D., Della Torre, A., Lacquaniti, A., *et al.* (2010) Neutrophil gelatinase-associated lipocalin levels in patients with Crohn disease undergoing treatment with infliximab. *Journal of Investigative Medicine*, **58**(3), 569–571.

3 Katz, L., Gisbert, J.P., Manoogian, B., *et al.* (2012) Doubling the infliximab dose versus halving the infusion intervals in Crohn's disease patients with loss of response. *Inflammatory Bowel Diseases*, **18**(11), 2026–2033.

4 Stein, D.J., Ananthakrishnan, A.N., Issa, M., *et al.* (2010) Impact of prior irregular infliximab dosing on performance of long-term infliximab maintenance therapy in Crohn's disease. *Inflammatory Bowel Diseases*, **16**(7), 1173–1179.

5 Farrell, R.J., Alsahli, M., Jeen, Y.T., *et al.* (2003) Intravenous hydrocortisone premedication reduces antibodies to infliximab in Crohn's disease: a randomized controlled trial. *Gastroenterology*, **124**(4), 917–924.

6 Rutgeerts, P., Sandborn, W.J., Feagan, B.G., *et al.* (2005) Infliximab for induction and maintenance therapy for ulcerative colitis. *New England Journal of Medicine*, **353**(23), 2462–2476.

7 Sandborn, W.J., Rutgeerts, P., Feagan, B.G., *et al.* (2009) Colectomy rate comparison after treatment of ulcerative colitis with placebo or infliximab. *Gastroenterology*, **137**(4), 1250–1260; quiz, 1520.

8 Colombel, J.F., Rutgeerts, P., Reinisch, W., *et al.* (2011) Early mucosal healing with infliximab is associated with improved long-term clinical outcomes in ulcerative colitis. *Gastroenterology*, **141**(4), 1194–1201.

9 Hyams, J., Damaraju, L., Blank, M., *et al.* (2012) Induction and maintenance therapy with infliximab for children with moderate to severe ulcerative colitis. *Clinical Gastroenterology and Hepatology*, **10**(4), 391–399.e1.

10 Sands, B.E., Tremaine, W.J., Sandborn, W.J., *et al.* (2001) Infliximab in the treatment of severe, steroid-refractory ulcerative colitis: a pilot study. *Inflammatory Bowel Diseases*, **7**(2), 83–88.

11 Jarnerot, G., Hertervig, E., Friis-Liby, I., *et al.* (2005) Infliximab as rescue therapy in severe to moderately severe ulcerative colitis: a randomized, placebo-controlled study. *Gastroenterology*, **128**(7), 1805–1811.

12 Gustavsson, A., Jarnerot, G., Hertervig, E., *et al.* (2010) Clinical trial: colectomy after rescue therapy in ulcerative colitis – 3-year follow-up of the Swedish–Danish controlled infliximab study. *Alimentary Pharmacology & Therapeutics*, **32**(8), 984–989.

13  van Dullemen, H.M., van Deventer, S.J., Hommes, D.W., *et al.* (1995) Treatment of Crohn's disease with anti-tumor necrosis factor chimeric monoclonal antibody (cA2). *Gastroenterology*, **109**(1), 129–135.

14  Targan, S.R., Hanauer, S.B., van Deventer, S.J., *et al.* (1997) A short-term study of chimeric monoclonal antibody cA2 to tumor necrosis factor alpha for Crohn's disease. Crohn's Disease cA2 Study Group. *New England Journal of Medicine*, **337**(15), 1029–1035.

15  Hanauer, S.B., Feagan, B.G., Lichtenstein, G.R., *et al.* (2002) Maintenance infliximab for Crohn's disease: the ACCENT I randomised trial. *Lancet*, **359**(9317), 1541–1549.

16  Rutgeerts, P., Diamond, R.H., Bala, M., *et al.* (2006) Scheduled maintenance treatment with infliximab is superior to episodic treatment for the healing of mucosal ulceration associated with Crohn's disease. *Gastrointestinal Endoscopy*, **63**(3), 433–442; quiz, 464.

17  Hanauer, S.B., Wagner, C.L., Bala, M., *et al.* (2004) Incidence and importance of antibody responses to infliximab after maintenance or episodic treatment in Crohn's disease. *Clinical Gastroenterology and Hepatology*, **2**(7), 542–553.

18  Baert, F., Noman, M., Vermeire, S., *et al.* (2003) Influence of immunogenicity on the long-term efficacy of infliximab in Crohn's disease. *New England Journal of Medicine*, **348**(7), 601–608.

19  Schnitzler, F., Fidder, H., Ferrante, M., *et al.* (2009) Long-term outcome of treatment with infliximab in 614 patients with Crohn's disease: results from a single-centre cohort. *Gut*, **58**(4), 492–500.

20  Gisbert, J.P. and Panes, J. (2009) Loss of response and requirement of infliximab dose intensification in Crohn's disease: a review. *American Journal of Gastroenterology*, **104**(3), 760–767.

21  Regueiro, M., Siemanowski, B., Kip, K.E., and Plevy, S. (2007) Infliximab dose intensification in Crohn's disease. *Inflammatory Bowel Diseases*, **13**(9), 1093–1099.

22  Chaparro, M., Martinez-Montiel, P., Van Domselaar, M., *et al.* (2012) Intensification of infliximab therapy in Crohn's disease: efficacy and safety. *Journal of Crohn's & Colitis*, **6**(1), 62–67.

23  Lin, K.K., Velayos, F., Fisher, E., and Terdiman, J.P. (2012) Durability of infliximab dose intensification in Crohn's disease. *Digestive Diseases and Sciences*, **57**(4), 1013–1019.

24  Vande Casteele, N., Khanna, R., Levesque, B.G., *et al.* (2015) The relationship between infliximab concentrations, antibodies to infliximab and disease activity in Crohn's disease. *Gut*, **64**(10), 1539–1545.

25  Afif, W., Leighton, J.A., Hanauer, S.B., *et al.* (2009) Open-label study of adalimumab in patients with ulcerative colitis including those with prior loss of response or intolerance to infliximab. *Inflammatory Bowel Diseases*, **15**(9), 1302–1307.

26  Van Assche, G., Magdelaine-Beuzelin, C., D'Haens, G., *et al.* (2008) Withdrawal of immunosuppression in Crohn's disease treated with scheduled infliximab maintenance: a randomized trial. *Gastroenterology*, **134**(7), 1861–1868.

27  Hyams, J., Crandall, W., Kugathasan, S., *et al.* (2007) Induction and maintenance infliximab therapy for the treatment of moderate-to-severe Crohn's disease in children. *Gastroenterology*, **132**(3), 863–873; quiz, 1165–1166.

28  Sands, B.E., Anderson, F.H., Bernstein, C.N., *et al.* (2004) Infliximab maintenance therapy for fistulizing Crohn's disease. *New England Journal of Medicine*, **350**(9), 876–885.

29  Sands, B.E., Blank, M.A., Patel, K., and van Deventer, S.J. (2004) Long-term treatment of rectovaginal fistulas in Crohn's disease: response to infliximab in the ACCENT II Study. *Clinical Gastroenterology and Hepatology*, **2**(10), 912–920.

30  Bouguen, G., Siproudhis, L., Gizard, E., *et al.* (2013) Long-term outcome of perianal fistulizing Crohn's disease treated with infliximab. *Clinical Gastroenterology and Hepatology*, **11**(8), 975–981.e1–4.

31  Moss, A.C., Fernandez-Becker, N., Jo Kim, K., *et al.* (2008) The impact of infliximab infusion reactions on long-term outcomes in patients with Crohn's disease. *Alimentary Pharmacology & Therapeutics*, **28**(2), 221–227.

32  Colombel, J.F., Loftus, E.V., Jr., Tremaine, W.J., *et al.* (2004) The safety profile of infliximab in patients with Crohn's disease: the Mayo Clinic experience in 500 patients. *Gastroenterology*, **126**(1), 19–31.

33  Lichtenstein, G.R., Rutgeerts, P., Sandborn, W.J., *et al.* (2012) A pooled analysis of infections, malignancy, and mortality in infliximab- and immunomodulator-treated adult patients with inflammatory bowel disease. *American Journal of Gastroenterology*, **107**(7), 1051–1063.

34  Grijalva, C.G., Chen, L., Delzell, E., *et al.* (2011) Initiation of tumor necrosis factor-alpha antagonists and the risk of hospitalization for infection in patients with autoimmune diseases. *JAMA*, **306**(21), 2331–2339.

35  Lichtenstein, G.R., Feagan, B.G., Cohen, R.D., *et al.* (2012) Serious infection and mortality in patients with Crohn's disease: more than 5 years of follow-up in the TREAT registry. *American Journal of Gastroenterology*, **107**(9), 1409–1422.

36  Ford, A.C. and Peyrin-Biroulet, L. (2013) Opportunistic infections with anti-tumor necrosis factor-alpha therapy in inflammatory bowel disease: meta-analysis of randomized controlled trials. *American Journal of Gastroenterology*, **108**(8), 1268–1276.

37  Hudesman, D., Lichtiger, S., and Sands, B. (2013) Risk of extraintestinal solid cancer with anti-TNF therapy in adults with inflammatory bowel disease: review of the literature. *Inflammatory Bowel Diseases*, **19**(3), 644–649.

38  Long, M.D., Martin, C.F., Pipkin, C.A., *et al.* (2012) Risk of melanoma and nonmelanoma skin cancer among patients with inflammatory bowel disease. *Gastroenterology*, **143**(2), 390–399.e1.

39  Chung, E.S., Packer, M., Lo, K.H., *et al.* (2003) Randomized, double-blind, placebo-controlled, pilot trial of infliximab, a chimeric monoclonal antibody to tumor necrosis factor-alpha, in patients with moderate-to-severe heart failure: results of the anti-TNF Therapy Against Congestive Heart Failure (ATTACH) trial. *Circulation*, **107**(25), 3133–3140.

40  Billioud, V., Sandborn, W.J., and Peyrin-Biroulet, L. (2011) Loss of response and need for adalimumab dose intensification in Crohn's disease: a systematic review. *American Journal of Gastroenterology*, **106**(4), 674–684.

41  Oussalah, A., Laclotte, C., Chevaux, J.B., *et al.* (2008) Long-term outcome of adalimumab therapy for ulcerative colitis with intolerance or lost response to infliximab: a single-centre experience. *Alimentary Pharmacology & Therapeutics*, **28**(8), 966–972.

42  Gies, N., Kroeker, K.I, Wong, K., and Fedorak, R.N. (2010) Treatment of ulcerative colitis with adalimumab or infliximab: long-term follow-up of a single-centre cohort. *Alimentary Pharmacology & Therapeutics*, **32**(4), 522–528.

43  Reinisch, W., Sandborn, W.J., Hommes, D.W., *et al.* (2011) Adalimumab for induction of clinical remission in moderately to severely active ulcerative colitis: results of a randomised controlled trial. *Gut*, **60**(6), 780–787.

44  Hanauer, S.B., Sandborn, W.J., Rutgeerts, P., *et al.* (2006) Human anti-tumor necrosis factor monoclonal antibody (adalimumab) in Crohn's disease: the CLASSIC-I trial. *Gastroenterology*, **130**(2), 323–333; quiz, 591.

45  Sandborn, W.J., Rutgeerts, P., Enns, R., *et al.* (2007) Adalimumab induction therapy for Crohn disease previously treated with

infliximab: a randomized trial. *Annals of Internal Medicine*, **146**(12), 829–838.

46 Colombel, J.F., Sandborn, W.J., Rutgeerts, P., *et al.* (2007) Adalimumab for maintenance of clinical response and remission in patients with Crohn's disease: the CHARM trial. *Gastroenterology*, **132**(1), 52–65.

47 Colombel, J.F., Sandborn, W.J., Rutgeerts, P., *et al.* (2009) Comparison of two adalimumab treatment schedule strategies for moderate-to-severe Crohn's disease: results from the CHARM trial. *American Journal of Gastroenterology*, **104**(5), 1170–1179.

48 Colombel, J.F., Schwartz, D.A., Sandborn, W.J., *et al.* (2009) Adalimumab for the treatment of fistulas in patients with Crohn's disease. *Gut*, **58**(7), 940–948.

49 Hyams, J.S., Griffiths, A., Markowitz, J., *et al.* (2012) Safety and efficacy of adalimumab for moderate to severe Crohn's disease in children. *Gastroenterology*, **143**(2), 365–374.e2.

50 Sandborn, W.J., Feagan, B.G., Stoinov, S., *et al.* (2007) Certolizumab pegol for the treatment of Crohn's disease. *New England Journal of Medicine*, **357**(3), 228–238.

51 Lichtenstein, G.R., Thomsen, O.O., Schreiber, S., *et al.* (2010) Continuous therapy with certolizumab pegol maintains remission of patients with Crohn's disease for up to 18 months. *Clinical Gastroenterology and Hepatology*, **8**(7), 600–609.

52 Sandborn, W.J., Schreiber, S., Hanauer, S.B., *et al.* (2010) Reinduction with certolizumab pegol in patients with relapsed Crohn's disease: results from the PRECiSE 4 Study. *Clinical Gastroenterology and Hepatology*, **8**(8), 696–702.e1.

53 Sandborn, W.J., Feagan, B.G., Marano, C., *et al.* (201) Subcutaneous golimumab induces clinical response and remission in patients with moderate to severe ulcerative colitis. *Gastroenterology*, **146**(1), 85–95; quiz, e14–15.

54 Sandborn, W.J., Feagan, B.G., Marano, C., *et al.* (2014) Subcutaneous golimumab maintains clinical response in patients with moderate-to-severe ulcerative colitis. *Gastroenterology*. **146**(1), 96–109.e1.

55 Ghosh, S., Goldin, E., Gordon, F.H., *et al.* (2003) Natalizumab for active Crohn's disease. *New England Journal of Medicine*, **348**(1), 24–32.

56 Sandborn, W.J., Colombel, J.F., Enns, R., *et al.* (2005) Natalizumab induction and maintenance therapy for Crohn's disease. *New England Journal of Medicine*, **353**(18), 1912–1925.

57 Feagan, B.G., Rutgeerts, P., Sands, B.E., *et al.* (2013) Vedolizumab as induction and maintenance therapy for ulcerative colitis. *New England Journal of Medicine*, **369**(8), 699–710.

58 Sandborn, W.J., Feagan, B.G., Rutgeerts, P., *et al.* (2013) Vedolizumab as induction and maintenance therapy for Crohn's disease. *New England Journal of Medicine*, **369**(8), 711–721.

59 Vermeire, S., O'Byrne, S., Keir, M., *et al.* (2014) Etrolizumab as induction therapy for ulcerative colitis: a randomised, controlled, phase 2 trial. *Lancet*, **384**(9940), 309–318.

60 Sandborn, W.J., Gasink, C., Gao, L.L., *et al.* (2012) Ustekinumab induction and maintenance therapy in refractory Crohn's disease. *New England Journal of Medicine*, **367**(16), 1519–1528.

61 Vuitton, L., Koch, S., and Peyrin-Biroulet, L. (2013) Janus kinase inhibition with tofacitinib: changing the face of inflammatory bowel disease treatment. *Current Drug Targets*, **14**(12), 1385–1391.

62 Axelrad, J., Bernheim, O., Colombel, J.F., *et al.* (2016) Risk of new or recurrent cancer in patients with inflammatory bowel disease and previous cancer exposed to immunosuppressive and anti-tumor necrosis factor agents. *Clinical Gastroenterology and Hepatology*, **14**(1), 58–64.

63 Colombel, J.F., Sandborn, W.J., Reinisch, W., *et al.* (2010) Infliximab, azathioprine, or combination therapy for Crohn's disease. *New England Journal of Medicine*, **362**(15), 1383–1395.

## Answers to Questions

1  Answer: **D**. Both psoriasis and lupus-like reactions are rare, immunologically mediated, adverse events that have been reported with infliximab, adalimumab, and certolizumab pegol in the treatment of Crohn's disease. A serum sickness-like reaction can occur following infliximab infusions and represents a delayed-type hypersensitivity reaction. Drug-induced systemic sclerosis has not been reported with anti-TNF agents.

2  Answer: **C**. Demyelinating neurologic disease, active untreated malignancy or infections, and decompensated heart failure represent absolute contraindications to use of anti-TNF agents. A personal history of solid organ malignancy was not associated with an increased risk of recurrence or new primaries in patients initiating biologic therapy [62]. A family history of Hodgkin's lymphoma is not associated with a significant increase in risk of immunosuppression-related lymphoma, which is usually of the non-Hodgkin's type.

3  Answer: **D**. Individuals who are seropositive for JC virus indicating prior exposure have an overall risk of PML of 1:1000 person-years, with this risk increasing even further to 1:100–1:500 after 2 years of use and in the setting of prior immunosuppressant use. In contrast to natalizumab, vedolizumab targets $\alpha_4\beta_7$, a gut-specific integrin, and has not been associated with increased risk of PML in exposed patients.

4  Answer: **B**. In the GEMINI clinical trials, co-treatment with immunomodulator therapy was not associated with higher rates of clinical response and remission compared with those on monotherapy with vedolizumab [57, 58].

# 9

## Antibiotics

---

### Clinical Take Home Messages

- Antibiotics are effective in the management of acute pouchitis in patients who have undergone total proctocolectomy and ileal pouch–anal anastomosis. Evidence supports the efficacy of both ciprofloxacin and metronidazole.
- There are limited data regarding the role of antibiotics in the management of luminal ulcerative colitis (UC) or Crohn's disease (CD). Data from randomized controlled trials suggest no benefit from

antimycobacterial treatment in the management of CD.
- Nitroimidazole antibiotics are effective in the prevention of postoperative recurrence in CD when taken for the first 3 months following resection. However, they may be poorly tolerated.
- There are no rigorous data supporting the efficacy of fecal microbiota transplantation in the management of UC or CD.

---

The intestinal microbiome and its interaction with the immune system play an important role in the pathogenesis of inflammatory bowel disease (IBD). In that context, there have been several therapeutic trials of antibiotics in the management of both ulcerative colitis (UC) and Crohn's disease (CD) for the treatment of active disease, maintenance of remission, and prevention of recurrence after resective surgery.

## Efficacy in Ulcerative Colitis

Few clinical trials have examined the role of antibiotics in the management of UC and have been heterogeneous, studying a spectrum of disease severity and varying in their

outcomes. Rahimi *et al.* performed a meta-analysis that included 530 patients enrolled in 10 randomized controlled trials (RCTs) [1]. The antibiotics studied included vancomycin, metronidazole, tobramycin, rifaximin, or a combination of other agents. Among the 263 patients randomized to antibiotics, 72% achieved clinical remission compared with 55% in the placebo group, yielding a pooled odds ratio of 2 in favor of antibiotic therapy. Subgroup analysis including only trials that examined short-term antibiotic treatment for 5–14 days revealed a similar effect in favor of antibiotic treatment. However, owing to the inconsistency in the antibiotics used, dose, and duration of therapy, and variations in definition of response, it is difficult to draw firm conclusions about

*Inflammatory Bowel Diseases: A Clinician's Guide*, First Edition. Ashwin N. Ananthakrishnan, Ramnik J. Xavier, and Daniel K. Podolsky.
© 2017 John Wiley & Sons Ltd. Published 2017 by John Wiley & Sons Ltd.

the efficacy of antibiotics in UC, particularly as some of the larger clinical trials included in the meta-analysis demonstrated no significant treatment effect. Acute severe colitis requiring hospitalization is a setting in which antibiotics are often used with the aim of reducing bacterial transmigration or preventing sepsis. In a trial of 39 patients with severe UC randomized to a combination of intravenous tobramycin and metronidazole or placebo, 63% of patients in the antibiotic group responded at 10 days compared with 65% in the placebo group [2]. In milder UC, oral tobramycin for 1 week as an adjunct to steroid therapy was more effective in achieving symptomatic remission than placebo [3]. No trials of antibiotics in UC have examined mucosal healing as an endpoint.

Antibiotics are frequently used for the treatment of pouchitis in patients who have undergone an ileal pouch–anal anastomosis after total proctocolectomy. Ciprofloxacin and metronidazole are the two most commonly used antibiotics. Shen *et al.* randomized 16 patients with acute pouchitis to a 2-week course of ciprofloxacin or metronidazole [4]. There was a significantly greater reduction in the pouch disease activity index in the group treated with ciprofloxacin than with metronidazole. One-third of patients in the metronidazole group developed adverse effects. The same antibiotics are effective in patients with recurrent or refractory pouchitis when used for 4 weeks [5], and sometimes as maintenance therapy in chronic refractory pouchitis [6]. Rifaximin may also have efficacy, although one study found a non-significant trend towards clinical remission compared with placebo at a dose of 1200 mg per day [7].

## Efficacy in Crohn's Disease

There are limited data addressing the role of antibiotics in the management of luminal CD disease. In a meta-analysis of 10 RCTs that examined the efficacy of antibiotics in inducing remission in 1160 patients with CD, antibiotics were more effective at inducing remission than placebo, although there was significant heterogeneity among the trials [8]. For example, a number of different antibiotic regimens were used in the trials, making it difficult to draw firm conclusions about the efficacy of any specific antibiotic. A single trial demonstrated efficacy of ciprofloxacin [9]. Trials of metronidazole and macrolides showed no efficacy. A multicenter phase 2 randomized trial found that use of rifaximin 800 mg twice daily was efficacious for the induction of remission in mild to moderate CD (62% vs. 43%) [10]. Addition of ciprofloxacin and metronidazole to budesonide therapy was associated with higher rates of remission in patients with colonic CD but not in those with small bowel disease, suggesting that the role of antibiotics in induction may depend on disease location [11].

Three trials also examined antibiotics as maintenance agents for the prevention of relapse, mostly antimycobacterial therapy for 9–12 months. Pooled data from the trials suggested a statistically significant effect of antibiotics in preventing CD relapse compared with placebo (RR 0.62, 95% CI 0.46–0.84), with a number needed to treat of 4. The variability in the interventions and patient populations precludes the possibility of drawing firm conclusions about the efficacy of antibiotics. Antibiotics are effective in the treatment of abscesses and perianal complications [12]. Ciprofloxacin and metronidazole are usually the first-line agents in that other broad-spectrum antibiotics such as amoxicillin/clavulanic acid or trimethoprim/sulfamethoxazole are also useful. The duration of antibiotic treatment varies based on clinical circumstances. Co-treatment with corticosteroids, immunomodulators, or anti-TNF biologics may be essential in the setting of significant luminal disease.

Considerable evidence supports the use of antibiotics in the prevention of postoperative recurrence. More than 80% of patients with CD develop disease recurrence. An initial trial supporting the role of antibiotics in preventing recurrence randomized 60 patients undergoing curative ileal resection to receive metronidazole daily for 3 months or placebo postoperatively [13]. At the end of week 12, 75% of patients in the placebo arm had recurrence compared with 52% of patients in the metronidazole group. Metronidazole also significantly reduced the risk of severe endoscopic recurrence, and clinical recurrence at 1 year. However, treatment was stopped in nearly one-third of patients in the metronidazole arm because of side effects. A second trial demonstrated ornidazole to be significantly superior to placebo in preventing clinical and endoscopic recurrence [14].

## Other Microbial Modification Methods – Probiotics and Fecal Microbiota Transplantation

There has been considerable interest in the modification of gut microbiota composition as a therapeutic approach. Several small studies have examined the efficacy of probiotics in CD. Most have been limited by small numbers of patients enrolled and the heterogeneity of the patient populations, concomitant treatments, and treatment endpoints. In a double-blind RCT of *Lactobacillus* GG in 75 patients with CD, there was no difference in remission between treatment and placebo [15]. A Cochrane systematic review including seven studies found no benefit from probiotics in maintaining medically or surgically induced remission in CD and only a statistically insignificant effect for the yeast *Saccharomyces boulardii* [16].

Evidence does support the efficacy of probiotics in UC but is limited to VSL#3 (a mixture of *Bifidobacterium breve, Bifidobacterium longum, Bifidobacterium infantis, Lactobacillus acidophilus, Lactobacillus plantarum, Lactobacillus paracasei, Lactobacillus bulgaricus*, and *Streptococcus thermophilus*). In several small studies of patients with mild to moderate UC, treatment with 3.6 billion colony forming units (CFU) of VSL#3 was associated with remission in 43% of patients compared with 16% in the placebo arm [17]. Two of the components of VSL#3 could be detected by polymerase chain reaction in colonic tissue biopsies on using 16S rRNA sequencing [18]. VSL#3 may also be effective in mild pouchitis [19]. There are no data supporting the efficacy of other probiotic preparations in UC.

With the promising efficacy of fecal microbiota transplantation (FMT) in *Clostridium difficile* colitis and increasing evidence supporting a central role for the microbiome in IBD pathogenesis, there is considerable interest in FMT as a treatment for IBD. However, the results so far have not been promising in either CD or UC, and have been limited by inconsistencies in study design, mode of delivery, number of treatments, patient population, and outcomes. Many patients express interest in FMT as a therapeutic option. However, the data supporting therapeutic efficacy of FMT in IBD have been limited to small, uncontrolled series with variable degrees of response and no control population. Among 18 studies, most of which were cohort studies or case series including 122 patients with either CD or UC, clinical remission was achieved in 45% of patients after FMT. However, there was a significant variation between the studies and the response rate was lower in UC (22%) than CD (61%) [20]. RCT of fecal transplantation in UC has been repeated and it failed to show a significant benefit compared with placebo after six weekly administrations via enema.

## Multiple Choice Questions

1   Which of the following antibiotics have demonstrated efficacy when used as adjunct to intravenous corticosteroids in acute severe ulcerative colitis?
    A  Ciprofloxacin and metronidazole.
    B  Tobramycin.
    C  Vancomycin.
    D  None of the above.

2   Which of the following antibiotics is associated with higher rates of remission in mild to moderate Crohn's disease?
    A  Rifaximin.
    B  Ciprofloxacin and metronidazole.
    C  Amoxicillin/clavulinic acid.
    D  None of the above.

3   Which of the following clinical scenarios is appropriate for the use of the probiotic VSL#3 in the management of IBD?
    A  Postoperative Crohn's disease for prevention of recurrence.
    B  Induction of remission in mild to moderate ileal Crohn's disease.
    C  Induction of remission in mild to moderate ulcerative colitis.
    D  Prevention of *C. difficile* infection in patients with inflammatory bowel disease receiving treatment with antibiotics.

# References

1 Rahimi, R., Nikfar, S., Rezaie, A., and Abdollahi, M. (2007) A meta-analysis of antibiotic therapy for active ulcerative colitis. *Digestive Diseases and Sciences*, **52**(11), 2920–2925.

2 Mantzaris, G.J., Hatzis, A., Kontogiannis, P., and Triadaphyllou, G. (1994) Intravenous tobramycin and metronidazole as an adjunct to corticosteroids in acute, severe ulcerative colitis. *American Journal of Gastroenterology*, **89**(1), 43–46.

3 Burke, D.A., Axon, A.T., Clayden, S.A., *et al.* (1990) The efficacy of tobramycin in the treatment of ulcerative colitis. *Alimentary Pharmacology & Therapeutics*, **4**(2), 123–129.

4 Shen, B., Achkar, J.P., Lashner, B.A., *et al.* (2001) A randomized clinical trial of ciprofloxacin and metronidazole to treat acute pouchitis. *Inflammatory Bowel Diseases*, **7**(4), 301–305.

5 Mimura, T., Rizzello, F., Helwig, U., *et al.* (2002) Four-week open-label trial of metronidazole and ciprofloxacin for the treatment of recurrent or refractory pouchitis. *Alimentary Pharmacology & Therapeutics*, **16**(5), 909–917.

6 Shen, B., Fazio, V.W., Remzi, F.H., *et al.* (2007) Combined ciprofloxacin and tinidazole therapy in the treatment of chronic refractory pouchitis. *Diseases of the Colon and Rectum*, **50**(4), 498–508.

7 Isaacs, K.L., Sandler, R.S., Abreu, M., *et al.* (2007) Rifaximin for the treatment of active pouchitis: a randomized, double-blind, placebo-controlled pilot study. *Inflammatory Bowel Diseases*, **13**(10), 1250–1255.

8 Khan, K.J., Ullman, T.A., Ford, A.C., *et al.* (2011) Antibiotic therapy in inflammatory bowel disease: a systematic review and meta-analysis. *American Journal of Gastroenterology*, **106**(4), 661–673.

9 Arnold, G.L., Beaves, M.R., Pryjdun, V.O., and Mook, W.J. (2002) Preliminary study of ciprofloxacin in active Crohn's disease. *Inflammatory Bowel Diseases*, **8**(1), 10–15.

10 Prantera, C., Lochs, H., Grimaldi, M., *et al.* (2012) Rifaximin-extended intestinal release induces remission in patients with moderately active Crohn's disease. *Gastroenterology*, **142**(3), 473–481.e4.

11 Steinhart, A.H., Feagan, B.G., Wong, C.J., *et al.* (2002) Combined budesonide and antibiotic therapy for active Crohn's disease: a randomized controlled trial. *Gastroenterology*, **123**(1), 33–40.

12 Thia, K.T., Mahadevan, U., Feagan, B.G., *et al.* (2009) Ciprofloxacin or metronidazole for the treatment of perianal fistulas in patients with Crohn's disease: a randomized, double-blind, placebo-controlled pilot study. *Inflammatory Bowel Diseases*, **15**(1), 17–24.

13 Rutgeerts, P., Hiele, M., Geboes, K., *et al.* (1995) Controlled trial of metronidazole treatment for prevention of Crohn's recurrence after ileal resection. *Gastroenterology*, **108**(6), 1617–1621.

14 Rutgeerts, P., Van Assche, G., Vermeire, S., *et al.* (2005) Ornidazole for prophylaxis of postoperative Crohn's disease recurrence: a randomized, double-blind, placebo-controlled trial. *Gastroenterology*, **128**(4), 856–861.

**15** Bousvaros, A., Guandalini, S., Baldassano, R.N., *et al.* (2005) A randomized, double-blind trial of *Lactobacillus* GG versus placebo in addition to standard maintenance therapy for children with Crohn's disease. *Inflammatory Bowel Diseases*, **11**(9), 833–839.

**16** Rolfe, V.E., Fortun, P.J., Hawkey, C.J., and Bath-Hextall, F. (2006) Probiotics for maintenance of remission in Crohn's disease. *Cochrane Database of Systematic Reviews*, (**4**), CD004826.

**17** Sood, A., Midha, V., Makharia, G.K., *et al.* (2009) The probiotic preparation, VSL#3 induces remission in patients with mild-to-moderately active ulcerative colitis. *Clinical Gastroenterology and Hepatology*, 7(11), 1202–1209.e1.

**18** Bibiloni, R., Fedorak, R.N., Tannock, G.W., *et al.* (2005) VSL#3 probiotic-mixture induces remission in patients with active ulcerative colitis. *American Journal of Gastroenterology*, **100**(7), 1539–1546.

**19** Gionchetti, P., Rizzello, F., Morselli, C., *et al.* (2007) High-dose probiotics for the treatment of active pouchitis. *Diseases of the Colon and Rectum*, **50**(12), 2075–2082; discussion, 2082–2084.

**20** Colman, R.J. and Rubin, D.T. (2014) Fecal microbiota transplantation as therapy for inflammatory bowel disease: a systematic review and meta-analysis. *Journal of Crohn's & Colitis*, **8**(12), 1569–1581.

**21** Gupta, V., Rodrigues, R., Nguyen, D., *et al.* (2016) Adjuvant use of antibiotics with corticosteroids in inflammatory bowel disease exacerbations requiring hospitalisation: a retrospective cohort study and meta-analysis. *Alimentary Pharmacology & Therapeutics*, **43**(1), 52–60.

## Answers to Questions

1  Answer: **D**. In small RCTs, addition of antibiotics to intravenous corticosteroid therapy in hospitalized patients with acute severe UC has not been associated with increased likelihood of clinical response or reduction in the likelihood of surgery [21].

2  Answer: **A**. A multicenter phase 2 randomized trial demonstrated efficacy of use of rifaximin 800 mg twice daily in the induction of remission in mild to moderate CD compared with placebo (62% vs. 43%) [10].

3  Answer: **C**. In several small studies of patients with mild to moderate UC, treatment with 3.6 billion CFU of VSL#3 was associated with remission in 43% of patients compared with 16% in the placebo arm [17]. There are no data demonstrating a role for VSL#3 in preventing *C. difficile* infection.

**Section III**

**Management**

# 10

# Medical Management of Ulcerative Colitis

## Clinical Take Home Messages

- The choice of therapy in ulcerative colitis (UC) is based on extent and severity of disease.
- The optimal treatment endpoint is resolution of symptoms, achievement of mucosal healing, and corticosteroid-free maintenance of remission.
- Limited colitis can be managed by either topical aminosalicylates alone or a combination or oral and topical aminosalicylates as first line.
- Approximately 30% of patients have extensive or pancolitis at presentation. Extensive disease requires oral therapy for induction and maintenance of remission. Oral aminosalicylates are first-line agents for mild to moderate pancolitis. Patients who do not respond to oral mesalamine within the first 2–4 weeks or are intolerant to mesalamine require corticosteroid therapy.
- Infliximab or infliximab and azathioprine in combination are more effective to achieve steroid-free remission in moderate to severe UC.
- Patients with severe UC require hospitalization for intravenous steroids, usually methylprednisone 40–60 mg per day administered in two or three divided doses or hydrocortisone 200–300 mg per day. Lack of response to steroids by day 3 is predictive of need for colectomy, and there is limited benefit to continuing intravenous steroids beyond 5–7 days without initiation of rescue therapy.
- Both infliximab and cyclosporine have similar short- and long-term efficacy in steroid-refractory UC.
- The surgery of choice in patients who are refractory to medical therapy is typically a total proctocolectomy with an ileal pouch–anal anastomosis (IPAA). This may be performed in two or three stages.

## Assessment of Extent, Activity, and Severity

The choice of therapy in ulcerative colitis (UC) is based on extent and severity of disease. For therapeutic decision-making and prognosis, patients can be stratified

as having proctitis or proctosigmoiditis, left-sided colitis, or extensive colitis. The transition from inflamed to non-inflamed mucosa in UC is often abrupt. However, it is important to sample tissue from both the inflamed and non-inflamed areas to define the histologic extent of the inflammation, as

*Inflammatory Bowel Diseases: A Clinician's Guide*, First Edition. Ashwin N. Ananthakrishnan, Ramnik J. Xavier, and Daniel K. Podolsky.
© 2017 John Wiley & Sons Ltd. Published 2017 by John Wiley & Sons Ltd.

this has implications for choice of therapy and also need for dysplasia surveillance.

There are several scales to stratify severity of UC. The Montreal system adopted a classification of S0–S3, with S0 representing clinical remission and lack of symptoms (see page 34). Mild UC is defined as the passage of four or fewer stools per day with or without blood, the absence of systemic illness, and normal inflammatory markers. Moderate UC is characterized as passage of more than four stools per day but with minimal signs of systemic toxicity. Severe UC is defined as passage of at least six bloody stools per day, tachycardia, fever, anemia, or elevated erythrocyte sedimentation rate [1]. The widely used Truelove and Witts classification of UC severity used similar definitions of mild, moderate, and severe disease, but also included a category of fulminant colitis defined by more than 10 bowel movements per day, continuous blood in the stool, fever, tachycardia, and requirement for transfusion (see page 35). In evaluating patients, it is useful to know the frequency of bowel movements and the proportion of the bowel movements that have visible blood. Several indices are available to assess disease activity in UC. The pediatric ulcerative colitis activity index (PUCAI) is one of the few that has been validated, and is also used to stratify disease severity in the Paris classification of pediatric UC. Another widely used index is the Mayo score, which comprises a clinical score and an endoscopic score including stool frequency, rectal bleeding, physician global assessment, and severity of endoscopic disease (Table 10.1).

In addition to ascertaining symptoms and features needed to assess severity of disease, a detailed medical history regarding potential triggers of relapse including medication, nonadherence, infections such as *Clostridium difficile*, and use of non-steroidal anti-inflammatory drugs (NSAIDs) should be obtained. History of recent initiation of medications that potentially trigger worsening of disease activity and intolerance or lack of response to

**Table 10.1** Components of the Mayo clinical and endoscopic scoring system in ulcerative colitis.

| Characteristic | Score |
| --- | --- |
| *Stool frequency (3-day average)* | |
| Normal number of stools | 0 |
| 1–2 stools per day more than normal | 1 |
| 3–4 stools per day more than normal | 2 |
| ≥5 stools per day more than normal | 3 |
| *Rectal bleeding* | |
| No blood seen | 0 |
| Streaks of blood seen with <50% of stools | 1 |
| Obvious blood seen with ≥50% of stools | 2 |
| Blood alone passed | 3 |
| *Physician global assessment* | |
| Normal | 0 |
| Mild disease | 1 |
| Moderate disease | 2 |
| Severe disease | 3 |
| *Findings on flexible sigmoidoscopy* | |
| Normal or inactive disease | 0 |
| Mild disease (erythema, decreased vascular pattern, mild friability) | 1 |
| Moderate disease (marked erythema, absent vascular pattern, friability, erosions) | 2 |
| Severe disease (spontaneous bleeding, ulceration) | 3 |

prior medical therapies are also important in therapeutic decision-making. Prior history of severe disease requiring hospitalization may be an important predictor of colectomy and is helpful in stratifying disease severity. Weight loss is another important objective marker of severe disease.

Thinking about the optimal treatment endpoint in UC is evolving. Resolution of symptoms is an important initial treatment goal, but several studies have demonstrated that attainment of mucosal healing may be associated with superior outcomes. Mucosal healing has usually been defined as a Mayo endoscopic subscore of 0 (normal) or 1 (mild disease). In the ACT trials, week 8 endoscopic healing was associated with better long-term clinical outcomes, including reduced risk of colectomy at week 52 [2]. The role of histologic healing in management is more unclear, as histologic changes may take longer to resolve than clinical features or endoscopic changes. Degree of histologic activity, assessed at a single point in time or over the cumulative history of disease, is predictive of risk of colorectal neoplasia [3]. The presence of acute inflammatory infiltrate and crypt abscesses was associated with higher rates of relapse [4]. However, there is no standard scoring system for grading histologic activity as none of the proposed scores have been validated [5].

## Limited Colitis – Proctitis, Proctosigmoiditis, and Left-sided Colitis

Topical agents are good for first line therapy in the management of ulcerative proctitis or proctosigmoiditis (Figure 10.1). Mesalamine suppositories 1000 mg nightly are a common first choice. In patients with refractory symptoms, suppositories should be used two or three times during the day. Mesalamine suppositories are more effective and safer than corticosteroid suppositories (hydrocortisone 25–30 mg daily) [6, 7]. The duration of treatment varies depending on the patient response. Once remission has been achieved, the interval between the suppositories can be lengthened and many patients are able to stop therapy altogether. Subsequent disease behavior can guide the need for maintenance therapy. Patients who are infrequent relapsers off therapy and whose disease flares respond quickly to initiation of topical treatment may be monitored for recurrence of symptoms with intermittent use of therapies during relapses. In contrast, patients who have persistent or frequent recurrent symptoms may benefit from maintenance mesalamine use [8]. Topical corticosteroids are an option for patients in whom disease does not respond to mesalamine suppositories or who have 5-aminosalicylic acid (5-ASA) intolerance. Systemic absorption of steroids

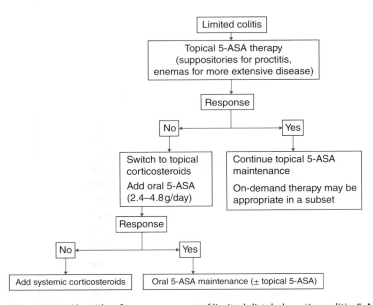

**Figure 10.1** Algorithm for management of limited distal ulcerative colitis. 5-ASA, 5-aminosalicylates.

with prolonged use is a concern, but this appears to be less a problem with suppositories than with enemas. There are limited data regarding the use of oral agents in the treatment of ulcerative proctitis, as most clinical trials exclude patients with isolated proctitis. In patients who are reluctant or unable to use topical therapy, oral mesalamine in doses for mild to moderate colitis may be initiated, although it is preferable to use this in conjunction with topical therapy when possible. Whether patients who achieve remission with topical therapy can be transitioned effectively to an oral therapy for maintenance has not been studied. Infrequently, patients with severe or refractory proctitis require escalation of therapy to systemic immunosuppression or biologic therapy.

As the reach of rectal suppositories is usually restricted to the rectum, patients with more proximal disease involving the sigmoid colon will benefit from use of a topical enema formulation or foam. The preferred first-line therapies are mesalamine enemas or foams administered nightly. After emptying the bladder, the patient instills the enemas and lies with their left side down for at least 30 minutes to ensure adequate coating of the affected areas. Many patients are able to retain the enemas the entire night. In patients with significant urgency who are not able to tolerate the enema formulation, foams are good alternatives; although they do not reach as high up in the colon as enemas, they may still achieve good topical efficacy and be better tolerated. Enemas can be used multiple times per day if needed, or used in combination with suppositories if the life style does not permit the use of enemas more than once per day. Topical mesalamine therapies may be used long term for maintenance with a low risk for relapse [9]. In patients who do not respond to or are intolerant to mesalamine enemas, hydrocortisone enemas or foam (Cortifoam®; 10% hydrocortisone foam) are good options.

Some patients with severe disease may tolerate these better than mesalamine enemas. Systemic absorption of corticosteroids and associated side effects with prolonged use can occur, making these a second-line option, and one used only infrequently for long-term maintenance.

Patients with left-sided UC often benefit from the use of topical therapies as outlined above. In patients with left-sided UC, combined therapy with oral 5-ASA along with topical therapy may be superior to oral mesalamine alone in the induction and maintenance of remission [10]. Long-term oral maintenance therapy is often better tolerated and preferred over topical treatment by patients. Some patients require infrequent (twice per week) use of enemas in addition to daily oral therapy in order to remain in remission. Corticosteroid enemas are an option for patients not achieving adequate response with oral and topical mesalamine therapy. Because of the estimated 40–80% systemic absorption with topical corticosteroid therapy, it is important to use these for the shortest duration possible and to transition to other oral or topical agents when possible. After extended topical hydrocortisone enema, therapy should not be stopped abruptly, to avoid precipitating adrenal insufficiency.

## Pancolitis

Approximately 30% of patients will have extensive colitis or pancolitis at presentation, and a subset of patients will be diagnosed with limited disease but evolve to develop pancolitis over the natural history of their disease. Extent of disease is an important predictor of natural history of disease, likelihood of eventual colectomy, and risk of colorectal cancer. Therapy for pancolitis depends on the severity of disease.

## Mild to Moderate Disease

Oral 5-aminosalicylates are the best first-line treatment for mild to moderate UC (Figure 10.2). Any of the oral 5-ASA agents are appropriate, with few available data from head-to-head comparisons of the different 5-ASA formulations. Sulfasalazine is less commonly used owing to cross-reaction with sulfa allergy and also non-allergenic side effects at the doses often required to achieve clinical remission. A head-to-head trial of balsalazide compared with mesalamine showed balsalazide to be more effective and better tolerated than mesalamine [11, 12]. An appropriate initial starting dose of mesalamine is 2.4 g per day or equivalent. Addition of topical 5-ASA or corticosteroids may provide quicker relief of troublesome distal symptoms. In patients with mild disease, there is no dose–response relationship between 2.4 and 4.8 g per day of mesalamine. However, in those with moderate disease, a 4.8 g per day dose achieves superior response compared with the 2.4 g per day dose. There are few data to suggest that patients who fail therapy with the 5-ASA compound achieve durable response to another agent within the same category.

Patients who do not respond to oral mesalamine within the first 2–4 weeks or are intolerant to mesalamine require corticosteroid therapy. Until recently, only systemically absorbed corticosteroids were available as a treatment option for UC. The availability of the budesonide multimatrix formulation (budesonide MMX®) with topical release throughout the entire colon including the left colon offers a promising and safer alternative in patients with mild or mild to moderate disease. Once patients have achieved remission with systemic steroids or the budesonide preparation, they should gradually taper the dose over the next 4–8 weeks. The pace of taper should be determined, in

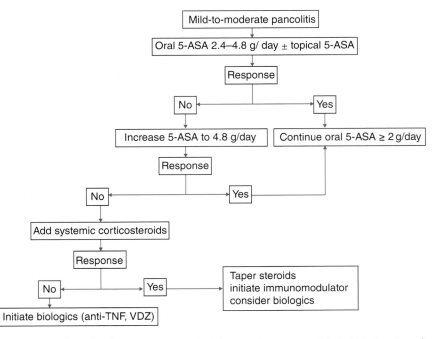

**Figure 10.2** Algorithm for management of mild-to-moderate pancolitis. 5-ASA, 5-aminosalicylates; anti-TNF, monoclonal antibodies to tumor necrosis factor alpha; VDZ, vedolizumab.

part, by the degree of response and also cumulative exposure to steroids over the course of their disease. Depending on disease severity, particularly when the patient is experiencing a first moderate flare of their disease despite a maintenance regimen, it may be appropriate to maintain them on their previous dose of mesalamine or to increase the dose to 4.8 g per day of mesalamine equivalent. However, in patients who have required two or more courses of corticosteroid therapy over a short period, escalation to immunosuppressive or biologic therapy should be strongly considered. Patients who are refractory to oral prednisone at a dose of 40 mg per day or equivalent may require hospitalization for intravenous corticosteroids and surgical evaluation.

Aminosalicylates are usually continued at the same dose during maintenance of remission. Although some patients who require 4.8 g per day of mesalamine or equivalent to achieve remission are able to reduce their dose back to 2.4 g per day, or 3.6 g per day for maintenance, in most patients the dose required for induction of remission is necessary for maintenance. A complete blood count, and also serum chemistry to monitor liver and renal function, should be obtained at least annually in patients on long-term aminosalicylate maintenance therapy. A urinalysis should be obtained every year to monitor for proteinuria due to interstitial nephritis. Corticosteroids are not optimal maintenance agents owing to a high risk of systemic side effects. Patients on long-term corticosteroids should have frequent monitoring of bone mineral density and daily supplementation with calcium and vitamin D.

### Moderate to Severe Disease

Patients with severe disease often require oral corticosteroids, typically in doses equivalent to 40–60 mg per day of prednisone. Patients should have laboratory testing to assess thiopurine methyltransferase (TPMT)

enzyme status and screening for latent tuberculosis and hepatitis B exposure in anticipation of starting systemic immunosuppression. Appropriate vaccination prior to the start of immunosuppression should be considered as the serologic response rates are higher. There are few comparative data between the different immunosuppressive agents in this setting. The UC SUCCESS trial compared conventional therapy using thiopurines with infliximab in patients with moderate to severe UC, defined as a Mayo score of 6 or higher, who were failing corticosteroid therapy and were either naive to azathioprine or had stopped it at least 3 months prior to the study [13]. At week 16, the primary endpoint of steroid-free remission was achieved in a larger proportion of patients in the infliximab–azathioprine combination arm (40%) than in those treated with only infliximab (22%) or azathioprine (24%). Clinical response and mucosal healing were also superior in the combined treatment arm compared with azathioprine. Thus preliminary evidence suggests that a biologic anti-TNF-based strategy may be more effective in patients with moderate to severe UC. However, the study duration of only 16 weeks was a major limitation of the trial. Long-term studies and also replication in other cohorts are essential prior to widespread adoption of early anti-TNF-based strategies in UC, particularly given the convenience of oral maintenance agents and the considerable difference in treatment costs between oral and biologic therapies. Clinical trial results indicate that adalimumab and golimumab are also effective treatment options for the management of moderate to severe UC. Vedolizumab has recently emerged as an attractive alternative for the management of such patients. The incremental benefit of vedolizumab over placebo appears to be superior to that of adalimumab in clinical trials, although the response rate for vedolizumab in patients with prior anti-TNF failure is inferior to that in patients who are anti-TNF naive [14].

Systemic immunosuppression may be lower with vedolizumab than with the anti-TNF agents, although long-term data are lacking. Patients who respond to an initial course of prednisone may be good candidates for thiopurine monotherapy, particularly in disease of moderate severity. Loss of response should trigger optimization of thiopurine dosing and ensure therapeutic drug levels and absence of shunting. Severe disease, lack of response to corticosteroids, intolerance, or failure of thiopurine therapy should prompt the use of biologic therapy (Figure 10.3). Both anti-TNF antibodies and vedolizumab are good options in this circumstance. with few data to guide the choice of one over the other. If a patient fails to respond to the first anti-TNF therapy, termed primary non-response, there is little likelihood of benefit from a second- or third-line anti-TNF agent and initiation of

an agent acting through an alternative mechanism of action, such as vedolizumab, should be considered. However, if a patient has initially responded to an anti-TNF agent, a loss of response may be overcome with a second-line anti-TNF biologic agent. Combination therapy with an immunomodulator (thiopurine or methotrexate) should be considered to reduce immunogenicity of the biologic drugs, boost response, and preserve durability.

Reduction of thiopurine dosage on achieving remission is not recommended. Patients who are long-term thiopurine users require continued monitoring of blood counts and liver function tests every 4 months, as leukopenia has been reported to occur even after several years of use with a stable dose. Patients should continue to be educated about immunosuppression-related side effects and advised to use appropriate preventive

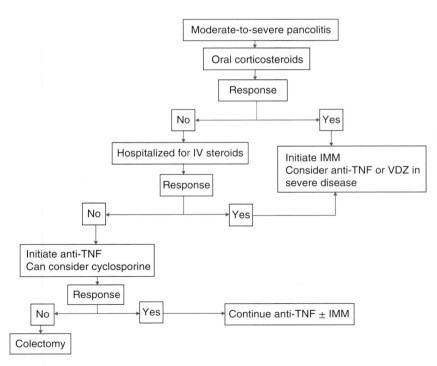

**Figure 10.3** Algorithm for management of moderate to severe UC. Anti-TNF, monoclonal antibodies to tumor necrosis factor alpha; VDZ, vedolizumab; IMM, immunomodulators.

measures such as wearing sunscreen and avoiding over-exposure to sunlight.

Similarly, a reduction in infliximab dose below $5\,\text{mg}\,\text{kg}^{-1}$ every 8 weeks is not advised. Every year, as many as 10–15% of patients lose response and require dose escalation. Increasing the dose or shortening the interval are equivalent in terms of efficacy. The availability of alternative anti-TNF agents and also the ability to perform therapeutic drug monitoring and identification of antidrug antibodies have offered further means to tailor its use. In patients who are not responding to infliximab, the first step involves establishing objective inflammation as a cause of the persistent symptoms. Then, a trough infliximab level and antibody status should be determined just prior to the next infusion. A subtherapeutic infliximab level ($<3\,\mu\text{g}\,\text{ml}^{-1}$) can be managed by increasing the dose. In patients who continue to have active inflammation despite therapeutic levels of infliximab, there is likely to be limited benefit to a trial of a second anti-TNF agent and an alternative mechanism of action should be initiated. In contrast, patients who lose response to infliximab because of antidrug antibodies may achieve a good response by switching to a different anti-TNF therapy.

### Severe Disease

Patients with severe UC should be hospitalized in order to receive supportive care and intravenous steroids, usually methylprednisone 40–60 mg per day administered in two or three divided doses or hydrocortisone 200–300 mg per day. Patients with new diagnosis of UC and recent initiation of 5-ASA therapy should have the medication stopped in consideration of possible drug-induced hypersensitivity. Patients may also benefit from topical hydrocortisone enemas for relief of distal symptoms. All patients should have a stool sample sent off to evaluate for infectious triggers, in particular *C. difficile* infection (Table 10.2). Empiric treatment of suspected *C. difficile* infection may be useful in a subgroup of patients while awaiting the results of the stool toxin assay. Hospitalized patients are at high risk for

Table 10.2 Stepwise management of acute severe colitis.

| | Stepwise management |
|---|---|
| 1 | Identify precipitants (infections such as *C. difficile*, CMV; non-adherence) |
| 2 | Low-fiber diet is appropriate for most patients. Nil-per-os if significant abdominal pain or vomiting. Antibiotics are not routinely indicated unless systemic signs |
| 3 | Minimize narcotics and anticholinergics |
| 4 | Prevent complications – venous thromboembolism prophylaxis |
| 5 | Flexible sigmoidoscopy for assessment of severity and biopsies for CMV infection |
| 6 | Initiate systemic steroids: 40–60 mg of prednisone equivalent. Add on local therapy as tolerated |
| 7 | Plan for next step in case of steroid refractoriness – obtain hepatitis B serology and testing for prior TB exposure; magnesium and lipid levels if considering cyclosporine |
| 8 | Objectively assess symptomatic and biochemical response on days 3 and 5 of intravenous steroid therapy |
| 9 | Early surgical consultation and co-management |
| 10 | If responding to inpatient treatment, optimize outpatient maintenance regimen to prevent future episodes |

venous thromboembolism and should receive thromboprophylaxis with unfractionated or low molecular weight heparins. These are usually safe even in the setting of overt rectal bleeding. Antibiotics have not been demonstrated to be effective in this setting, but some practitioners initiate such therapy if fever or other systemic signs are present. Early surgical consultation and co-management with surgeons are important in caring for a patient with severe disease requiring hospitalization. The management of pain in patients with acute severe colitis is challenging. The use of narcotics should be avoided owing to the possibility of precipitating toxic megacolon. Anticholinergics should also be avoided for the same reason. Close monitoring of nutritional status is essential, as low albumin is associated with inferior response to medical therapy and also more complications after surgery.

Although most patients are initially kept nil-per-os, the diet can be gradually advanced to a low-residue diet as tolerated. Patients with abdominal pain should have at least a plain film of the abdomen to rule out toxic megacolon or free perforation. Small intestinal air content may be predictive of subsequent development of toxic megacolon or need for colectomy. Patients with systemic signs may require a computed tomography (CT) scan to rule out extraluminal complications or subtle microperforation. On admission, it is important to obtain a lipid panel and a magnesium level, in addition to screening for prior hepatitis B and tuberculosis exposure so that either infliximab or cyclosporine therapy can be initiated without delay in case of non-response to steroids. The role of early endoscopic evaluation in this setting has been debated. Early endoscopy allows for assessment of severity of disease which carries prognostic significance. Furthermore, sigmoidoscopy allows biopsies o be obtained for diagnosis of cytomegalovirus infection.

Lack of response to steroids by day 3 is predictive of need for colectomy. About 85% of patients who had more than eight stools or had between three and eight stools and a C-reactive protein (CRP) level of 45 mg l$^{-1}$ or higher have required colectomy [15]. There is limited benefit to continuing intravenous steroids beyond 5–7 days without initiation of rescue therapy. In patients who are thiopurine naive, either infliximab or cyclosporine is an appropriate option, with similar times to response and similar short-term outcomes [16]. In patients who have failed thiopurine therapy as outpatients, infliximab is the preferred choice as it allows for continuation as a maintenance agent if the disease responds. There are limited data on therapeutic drug monitoring in the acute setting to guide timing of subsequent dosing if there is incomplete response to the first dose of infliximab. Infliximab and cyclosporine have each been used as rescue therapy in the setting of failure of the other agent; however, success has been modest, with a significant incidence of infectious complications [17, 18]. There are no data on the effectiveness of adalimumab, golimumab, or vedolizumab in the setting of the hospitalized severe UC patient.

The surgery of choice in patients who are refractory to medical therapy is typically a subtotal colectomy with an ileostomy and a Hartmann's pouch. A three-stage approach can be adopted, with subsequent proctectomy and J-pouch creation as a second stage, and closure of ileostomy as the third stage. It is uncertain whether preoperative biologic therapy influences risk of postoperative infections. However, in patients with refractory or fulminant disease, exposure to biologic therapy should not lead to a delay in appropriate surgical treatment. Fulminant colitis and toxic megacolon are indications for emergency surgery. Patients who achieve incomplete response to medical therapy remain at high risk for relapse and colectomy and should be closely followed after discharge from hospital with early up-titration of medical regimen.

# Case Studies and Multiple Choice Questions

1   Juan is a 23-year-old financial analyst who has a 4-month history of four bowel movements daily, one nocturnal bowel movement per week, urgency, and tenesmus, with visible blood in approximately one-third of the bowel movements. He has a family history of ulcerative colitis in two maternal cousins. He denies any travel or recent antibiotic use. You perform a colonoscopy, which reveals pancolitis of moderate severity (Mayo 2). Which of the following treatments is appropriate for initial management of Juan?
   A   Start oral mesalamine 2.4 g daily.
   B   Start oral mesalamine 2.4 g daily in conjunction with mesalamine retention enemas.
   C   Start anti-TNF biologic therapy.
   D   Start prednisone 60 mg daily.

2   Two months later, Juan returns to your office having been on oral mesalamine 2.4 g daily and mesalamine enemas at night. He reports no improvement in symptoms with still five bowel movements per day and one nocturnal bowel movement per week. He is still seeing visible blood at least 30% of the time. He assures you of full compliance with therapy and denies any recent NSAID use. Which of the following is the most appropriate next step?
   A   Add ciprofloxacin and metronidazole for 2 weeks.
   B   Start anti-TNF biologic therapy.

   C   Start azathioprine 2.5 mg kg$^{-1}$ daily.
   D   Increase the dose of mesalamine to 4.8 g daily.

3   Audrey is a 22-year-old woman diagnosed with ulcerative colitis 6 months earlier. She was started on treatment with mesalamines and, after no response, initiated oral prednisone 1 month ago. Owing to persistent symptoms on 40 mg per day of oral prednisone, she was admitted to the hospital and started on methylprednisolone 60 mg intravenously daily. After 7 days of therapy, her condition was unchanged and she continued to have 10 bowel movements per day, all of which were grossly bloody. She also is experiencing continued tenesmus and abdominal cramping. Physical examination reveals normal bowel sounds and mild left lower quadrant tenderness without rebound or guarding. Laboratory findings suggest a hemoglobin of 10.1 g dl$^{-1}$, albumin of 3.2 g dl$^{-1}$ and CRP of 83 mg dl$^{-1}$. Which of the following is an appropriate next step in her care?
   A   Perform a CT scan of the abdomen to look for extent of colitis and abdominal abscess formation.
   B   Perform an unprepped flexible sigmoidoscopy with biopsies.
   C   Perform a complete colonoscopy with ileal examination and cytomegalovirus (CMV) antigenemia assay.
   D   Perform magnetic resonance enterography (MRE).

4   A flexible sigmoidoscopy is performed on Audrey and reveals severe inflammation (Mayo 3) in the rectum, sigmoid colon, and descending colon. Biopsies confirm severe colitis and do not show any evidence of CMV infection. Which of the following is the best next step in Audrey's care?

A   Continue intravenous corticosteroids for a further 7 days.

B   Keep her nil-per-os and initiate intravenous antibiotics and parenteral nutrition.

C   Initiate rescue therapy with infliximab or cyclosporine.

D   Initiate rescue therapy with vedolizumab.

5   You decide to initiate therapy with infliximab or cyclosporine. Which of the following statements about rescue therapy is true?

A   Audrey is not a candidate for cyclosporine because of her age and gender, as cyclosporine is contraindicated in women of childbearing age.

B   Both infliximab and cyclosporine are equally likely to result in response and have similar time to response and reduction in risk of colectomy.

C   Hypercholesterolemia and hypermagnesemia represent relative contraindications to the use of cyclosporine.

D   Since she is thiopurine naive, Audrey is likely to have worse outcomes after initiation of cyclosporine.

# References

1 Satsangi, J., Silverberg, M.S., Vermeire, S., and Colombel, J.F. (2006) The Montreal classification of inflammatory bowel disease: controversies, consensus, and implications. *Gut*, **55**(6), 749–753.

2 Colombel, J.F., Rutgeerts, P., Reinisch, W., *et al.* (2011) Early mucosal healing with infliximab is associated with improved long-term clinical outcomes in ulcerative colitis. *Gut*, **141**(4), 1194–1201.

3 Rubin, D.T., Huo, D., Kinnucan, J.A., *et al.* (2013) Inflammation is an independent risk factor for colonic neoplasia in patients with ulcerative colitis: a case–control study. *Clinical Gastroenterology and Hepatology*, **11**(12), 1601–1608.e1–4.

4 Riley, S.A., Mani, V., Goodman, M.J., *et al.* (1991) Microscopic activity in ulcerative colitis: what does it mean? *Gut*, **32**(2), 174–178.

5 Peyrin-Biroulet, L., Bressenot, A., and Kampman, W. (2014) Histologic remission: the ultimate therapeutic goal in ulcerative colitis? *Clinical Gastroenterology and Hepatology*, **12**(6), 929–934.e2.

6 Lucidarme, D., Marteau, P., Foucault, M., *et al.* (1997) Efficacy and tolerance of mesalazine suppositories vs. hydrocortisone foam in proctitis. *Alimentary Pharmacology & Therapeutics*, **11**(2), 335–340.

7 Cohen, R.D., Woseth, D.M., Thisted, R.A., and Hanauer, S.B. (2000) A meta-analysis and overview of the literature on treatment options for left-sided ulcerative colitis and ulcerative proctitis. *American Journal of Gastroenterology*, **95**(5), 1263–1276.

8 Marteau, P., Crand, J., Foucault, M., and Rambaud, J.C. (1998) Use of mesalazine slow release suppositories 1 g three times per week to maintain remission of ulcerative proctitis: a randomised double blind placebo controlled multicentre study. *Gut*, **42**(2), 195–199.

9 Ford, A.C., Khan, K.J., Sandborn, W.J., *et al.* (2012) Efficacy of topical 5-aminosalicylates in preventing relapse of quiescent ulcerative colitis: a meta-analysis. *Clinical Gastroenterology and Hepatology*, **10**(5), 513–519.

10 Ford, A.C., Khan, K.J., Achkar, J.P., and Moayyedi, P. (2012) Efficacy of oral vs. topical, or combined oral and topical 5-aminosalicylates, in ulcerative colitis: systematic review and meta-analysis. *American Journal of Gastroenterology*, **107**(2), 167–176; author reply, 177.

11 Green, J.R., Lobo, A.J., Holdsworth, C.D., *et al.* (1998) Balsalazide is more effective and better tolerated than mesalamine in the treatment of acute ulcerative colitis. The Abacus Investigator Group. *Gastroenterology*, **114**(1), 15–22.

12 Pruitt, R., Hanson, J., Safdi, M., *et al.* (2002) Balsalazide is superior to mesalamine in the time to improvement of signs and symptoms of acute mild-to-moderate ulcerative colitis. *American Journal of Gastroenterology*, **97**(12), 3078–3086.

13 Panaccione, R., Ghosh, S., Middleton, S., *et al.* (2014) Combination therapy with

infliximab and azathioprine is superior to monotherapy with either agent in ulcerative colitis. *Gastroenterology*, **146**(2), 392–400.e3.

14  Sands, B.E., Feagan, B.G., Rutgeerts, P., *et al.* (2014) Effects of vedolizumab induction therapy for patients with Crohn's disease in whom tumor necrosis factor antagonist treatment failed. *Gastroenterology*, **147**(3), 618–627.e3.

15  Travis, S.P., Farrant, J.M., Ricketts, C., *et al.* (1996) Predicting outcome in severe ulcerative colitis. *Gut*, **38**(6), 905–910.

16  Laharie, D., Bourreille, A., Branche, J., *et al.* (2012) Ciclosporin versus infliximab in patients with severe ulcerative colitis refractory to intravenous steroids: a parallel, open-label randomised controlled trial. *Lancet*, **380**(9857), 1909–1915.

17  Chang, K.H., Burke, J.P., and Coffey, J.C. (2013) Infliximab versus cyclosporine as rescue therapy in acute severe steroid-refractory ulcerative colitis: a systematic review and meta-analysis. *International Journal of Colorectal Disease*, **28**(3), 287–293.

18  Maser, E.A., Deconda, D., Lichtiger, S., *et al.* (2008) Cyclosporine and infliximab as rescue therapy for each other in patients with steroid-refractory ulcerative colitis. *Clinical Gastroenterology and Hepatology*, **6**(10), 1112–1116.

19  Hanauer, S.B., Sandborn, W.J., Kornbluth, A., *et al.* (2005) Delayed-release oral mesalamine at 4.8 g/day (800 mg tablet) for the treatment of moderately active ulcerative colitis: the ASCEND II trial. *American Journal of Gastroenterology*, **100**(11), 2478–2485.

20  Carbonnel, F., Boruchowicz, A., Duclos, B., *et al.* (1996) Intravenous cyclosporine in attacks of ulcerative colitis: short-term and long-term responses. *Digestive Diseases and Sciences*, **41**(12), 2471–2476.

21  Arts, J., D'Haens, G., Zeegers, M., *et al.* (2004) Long-term outcome of treatment with intravenous cyclosporin in patients with severe ulcerative colitis. *Inflammatory Bowel Diseases*, **10**(2), 73–78.

## Answers to Questions

1   Answer: **B.** Aminosalicylates are first-line therapy for induction of remission in patients with mild to moderate ulcerative colitis. In a systematic review, combined therapy with topical and oral 5-ASAs was superior to oral 5-ASA alone for induction of remission and should be the preferred strategy, particularly in patients with significant distal symptoms [10].

2   Answer: **D.** In the ASCEND clinical trial, for milder ulcerative colitis, both 2.4 and 4.8 g per day of mesalamine appear to have comparable efficacy for induction of remission (51% vs. 56%). In contrast, for those with moderate disease, there is a higher likelihood of response with the 4.8 g per day dose (72%) than the 2.4 g per day dose (57%) [19]. Consequently, the best next step for Juan would be to optimize his aminosalicylates dose by increasing it to 4.8 g per day.

3   Answer: **B.** Audrey has steroid refractory acute severe colitis. Up to one-third of patients with steroid refractory ulcerative colitis may have CMV colitis complicating their disease. Reliable diagnosis of CMV colitis can only be established by obtaining biopsies from an inflamed segment of the colon and subjecting them to either viral culture or immunohisto-chemistry. CMV antigenemia has poor sensitivity and specificity in diagnosing CMV colitis. Additionally, a complete colonoscopy is associated with higher risk of perforation in acutely ill patients and a sigmoidoscopy is usually sufficient to establish a diagnosis. There is no suspicion for extraluminal complications in Audrey and consequently a CT scan or MRE is not required.

4   Answer: **C.** Audrey has steroid refractory acute severe colitis. There is limited benefit to continuing intravenous corticosteroids beyond 5–10 days. Early initiation of rescue therapy should be considered in patients who have more than eight bowel movements or between three and eight bowel movements and CRP >45 mg l$^{-1}$ after 3 days of intravenous corticosteroids [15]. Studies have also demonstrated no benefit to total parenteral nutrition (TPN) in patients with acute severe colitis. Vedolizumab is effective in inducing and maintaining remission in ulcerative colitis but has not been studied in the setting of acute severe colitis. Hence rescue therapy should be initiated with infliximab or cyclosporine, which are the only two agents with established efficacy in this setting.

5   Answer: **B.** In the large, randomized CYSIF trial comparing infliximab and cyclosporine in the management of acute severe colitis, there were similar rates of treatment failure (60% vs. 54%) in patients

receiving infliximab and cyclosporine [16]. Hypocholesterolemia and hypomagnesemia represent relative contraindications to the use of cyclosporine owing to increased risk of seizures. Patients who are thiopurine naive are likely to have superior outcomes with use of cyclosporine and initiation of thiopurines on discharge from the hospital than patients with prior thiopurine failure [20, 21]. Cyclosporine is not associated with increased risk of birth defects and is not contraindicated in women of childbearing age.

# 11

# Medical Management of Crohn's Disease

## Clinical Take Home Messages

- The key factors determining treatment of Crohn's disease (CD) are disease location, behavior, and potential for disease progression.
- Early effective therapy in CD is key to improving long-term outcomes and avoiding progressive bowel damage.
- Aminosalicylates are usually not effective in the management of CD but may be useful in a subset of patients with very mild disease. Budesonide is an effective alternative to systemic corticosteroids in the induction of remission in mild to moderate ileocolonic CD.
- Owing to the delay in the onset of action, azathioprine or 6-mercaptopurine are not effective as a sole induction agent but they have demonstrated benefit in maintenance of remission and reduction of the need for corticosteroids.
- A combination of azathioprine and an anti TNF or anti TNF alone is superior to azathioprine in patients with recent diagnosis of CD who are naive to immunomodulator therapy.

There is substantial overlap between the principles of management of ulcerative colitis (UC) and Crohn's disease (CD). The key factors determining treatment of CD are disease location, behavior, and potential for disease progression. Most patients are diagnosed with the inflammatory phenotype of CD. With progressively longer duration of disease, it evolves into fistulizing or stricturing phenotypes. As both of these are associated with higher rates or surgery and lower rates of response to medical therapy, effective therapy early on in the course of CD is important to prevent the development of these complications.

The optimal therapeutic endpoint in CD, as in UC, remains a moving target. Although symptom-based disease activity indices such as the Crohn's disease activity index (CDAI) are commonly used to define treatment response in clinical trials, it is well recognized that symptoms correlate poorly with objective markers of inflammation [1]. There is increasing focus on mucosal healing as the therapeutic endpoint. Trials of all three available anti-tumor necrosis factor (TNF) biologics and vedolizumab have demonstrated that it is possible to achieve mucosal healing. Furthermore, mucosal healing is associated with a reduced need for

*Inflammatory Bowel Diseases: A Clinician's Guide*, First Edition. Ashwin N. Ananthakrishnan, Ramnik J. Xavier, and Daniel K. Podolsky.
© 2017 John Wiley & Sons Ltd. Published 2017 by John Wiley & Sons Ltd.

steroids, higher rates of clinical response, and lower rates of surgery on maintenance therapy [2, 3]. The cost of dose escalation to achieve mucosal healing may be offset by subsequent cost savings in hospitalization and surgeries, making it a cost-effective therapeutic endpoint from a societal perspective [4].

Recent evidence supports the importance of early effective therapy in CD to improve long-term outcomes and avoid progressive bowel damage. Patients with early CD have higher rates of response to biologic therapy than those with established disease. A subgroup analysis of the PRECISE 3 trial showed higher rates of response and remission in patients within 1 year of disease compared with those with disease duration of 5 years or longer. To examine rigorously the concept of early therapy, D'Haens *et al.* randomized patients to one of two strategies [5]. In the conventional strategy arm, patients received treatment with azathioprine after failure of corticosteroid therapy. If patients relapsed on azathioprine, they were treated with infliximab. In contrast, in the early combined immunosuppression strategy, patients received a loading dose of infliximab up front along with azathioprine, with reintroduction of infliximab for subsequent disease flares. At weeks 26 and 52, patients in the early combined treatment arm had higher rates of steroid-free clinical remission without surgical resection compared with placebo. In addition, at 2 years, patients in the early combined treatment arm had higher rates of mucosal healing.

Several factors may contribute to symptoms in patients with CD, not all of them being attributable to active disease. The first step in the management is to establish whether symptoms are related to active inflammatory disease and are not due to fibrostenotic complications or other comorbidities. A substantial proportion of patients with CD continue to have irritable bowel syndrome-like symptoms while in remission [6]; therapy escalation is both inappropriate and ineffective in that circumstance. Patients who have had ileocecal resection may have bile acid malabsorption leading to coleretic diarrhea that can typically be managed by bile acid-binding resins. Short bowel syndrome can contribute to diarrhea in patients who have extensive disease or after multiple bowel resections; bile acid-binding resins typically worsen diarrhea in such settings and should be avoided. Diarrhea can also occur due to "dumping" from the loss of the "ileal brake" phenomenon after ileocecal resection, or due to coexisting conditions such as *Clostridium difficile* infection, celiac disease, or small intestinal bacterial overgrowth.

## Mild to Moderate Disease

The role of aminosalicylates in the management of mild to moderate CD remains controversial, with most clinical trials showing at best modest efficacy in maintaining remission. However, a subgroup of patients, particularly those with colonic CD, may respond to mesalamine-based agents. Patients with ileal CD may benefit from agents that are not dependent on pH for release of the aminosalicylate moiety such as the moisture-release agent mesalamine (Pentasa). Despite a lack of supporting data, these agents are commonly used as first-line therapy for mild CD. However, recognizing the lack of efficacy, it is important to move on early to more effective treatments in the setting of non-response or relapse. There are also few data supporting the role of antibiotics as induction or maintenance agents for mild to moderate CD. However, a fairly recent trial did demonstrate rifaximin to be effective for inducing remission in moderate disease [7].

Budesonide is an effective alternative for the induction of remission in mild to moderate CD involving the ileum and right colon.

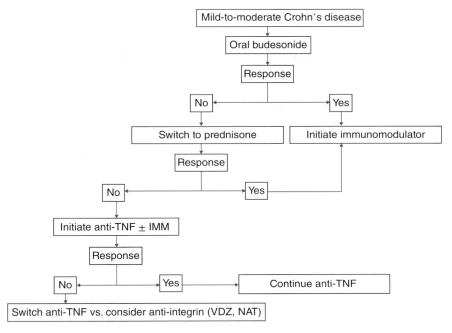

**Figure 11.1** Algorithm for management of mild-to-moderate CD. Anti-TNF, monoclonal antibodies to tumor necrosis factor alpha; VDZ, vedolizumab; NAT, natalizumab; IMM, immunomodulator.

It is typically initiated in doses of 9 mg once per day for 8–12 weeks, followed by a taper by 3 mg per day every few weeks (Figure 11.1). Budesonide 6 mg per day was not effective as maintenance therapy beyond 6 months. Budesonide is less effective than prednisone, which may be better for patients with moderate disease, if patients do not respond to budesonide therapy, or if they have pancolonic disease. Patients on budesonide or prednisone should be monitored closely for steroid-related side effects.

Owing to the delay in the onset of action, azathioprine or 6-mercaptopurine is not effective as a sole induction agent except in patients with very mild symptoms. They are usually initiated in doses of 50 mg per day of azathioprine or 25–50 mg per day of 6-mercaptopurine after confirming normal thiopurine methyltransferase (TPMT) enzyme activity (or with a reduced dose in those with intermediate enzyme activity), with escalation up to the target dose within 4–6

weeks in conjunction with frequent blood count monitoring. Methotrexate is also an effective option for both the induction and maintenance of remission in CD of moderate severity. The induction dose of methotrexate is 25 mg administered subcutaneously or intramuscularly every week along with folic acid supplementation for 12–16 weeks. After achievement of clinical remission, the dose is reduced to 15 mg weekly, but some patients may require a higher dose for maintenance.

## Moderate to Severe Disease

Most patients with moderate to severe CD require immunomodulator or biologic therapy, although the threshold for initiation of biologic therapy remains a matter of clinical judgment (Figure 11.2). The SONIC trial demonstrated that a combination of azathioprine and infliximab or infliximab alone

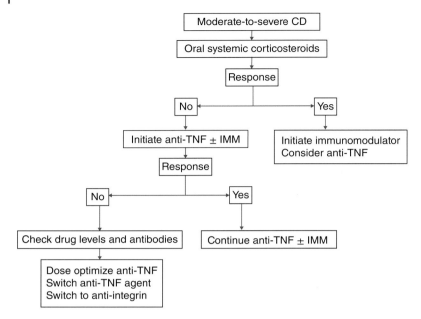

**Figure 11.2** Algorithm for management of moderate-to severe CD. Anti-TNF, monoclonal antibodies to tumor necrosis factor alpha; IMM, immunomodulator.

was superior to azathioprine in patients with recent diagnosis of CD who were naive to immunomodulator therapy. However, in clinical practice, there is a subgroup of patients with CD who respond well and remain in remission on thiopurines. In addition, given the substantial treatment costs and sometimes circumscribed durability of biologic therapy, patients with moderate disease and no risk factors that suggest early progression to penetrating disease or need for surgery may be tried on thiopurine as first-line therapy. Patients with risk factors suggesting aggressive disease such as perianal fistulizing disease, extensive or upper gastrointestinal involvement, early age of diagnosis, need for multiple courses of corticosteroids, or penetrating disease should begin biologic therapy early.

There have been no head-to-head comparative trials to guide choice of biologic agent. Randomized controlled trials suggest comparable benefits over placebo in trials of each of the anti-TNF antibodies. Patient

convenience is often a determining factor, particularly in those with luminal CD. Patients with high-risk phenotypes outlined above may benefit from early combination therapy. Many practitioners advocate long-term low-dose combination therapy to reduce immunogenicity, although there is little evidence in support of a low-dose versus a standard-dose combination therapy strategy. The low-dose strategy may be adopted in individuals at higher risk for complications from combination therapy, such as young males who are more likely to develop hepatosplenic T-cell lymphoma.

The first step in the management of patients who lose a previous response to the first anti-TNF therapy is to determine whether their symptoms are from objective inflammation, fibrostenotic complications, or functional comorbidity. As discussed for UC in Chapter 10, measurement of trough drug levels and antidrug antibodies may be useful in guiding subsequent therapy. Patients with undetectable levels of infliximab at trough may expect a good response with dose escalation. In contrast, patients losing response due to antidrug antibodies are likely not to benefit from dose escalation. However, anecdotal reports suggest that antidrug antibodies may be transient [8] or may resolve with escalation of dose or addition of immunomodulator therapy [9]. Since antidrug antibodies are not cross-reactive between the different anti-TNF agents, patients losing response due to such antibodies usually respond well to a second anti-TNF agent. There may be a small incremental benefit to a third anti-TNF agent in the setting of two prior anti-TNF failures, although the durability of this is usually limited [10, 11]. Patients with objective inflammation despite adequate levels of infliximab at trough usually exhibit poor incremental response with another anti-TNF agent and instead benefit from a switch to a different class of therapy such as vedolizumab. Vedolizumab has emerged as an attractive option for use in patients who are primary non-responders to anti-TNF biologic therapy in CD, and as a third-line agent in those with secondary loss of response to anti-TNF antibodies. The delayed onset of action (~10 weeks after initiation) makes this less suitable in patients with severe or steroid-refractory disease. In severe refractory CD, tacrolimus and mycophenolate have demonstrated efficacy in small series.

# Case Studies and Multiple Choice Questions

1  Monica is a 27-year-old woman with a 5-year history of Crohn's disease who initiated therapy with infliximab 5 mg kg$^{-1}$ at weeks 0, 2, and 6 followed by maintenance infusions every 8 weeks. She had previously been on therapy with mesalamine 4.8 g daily and azathioprine 125 mg per day (2.5 mg kg$^{-1}$) without adequate response and requiring repeated courses of prednisone. She has a good response to infliximab with normal bowel movements and cessation of diarrhea and abdominal pain after the first three doses. Twelve months after initiation of therapy with infliximab, she develops diarrhea, rectal bleeding, and weight loss. A colonoscopy is performed and reveals moderate active disease throughout the colon. Which of the following is the best next step to optimize her therapy?

A  Increase infliximab to 10 mg kg$^{-1}$ every 4 weeks.

B  Add prednisone 40 mg per day and continue infliximab 5 mg kg$^{-1}$ every 8 weeks.

C  Label her a primary non-responder to infliximab and switch to vedolizumab.

D  Obtain infliximab trough levels and antidrug antibodies.

2  You obtain drug levels and antibodies at trough (just prior to next infusion). This reveals no anti-infliximab antibodies and a trough level of 7 µg ml$^{-1}$. Which is the best next step in Monica's treatment?

A  Increase the infliximab dose to 10 mg kg$^{-1}$ every 4 weeks.

B  Stop infliximab and switch to adalimumab.

C  Stop infliximab and switch to vedolizumab.

D  Add ciprofloxacin and metronidazole for 1 month.

3  Kevin is a 20-year-old man with a family history of Crohn's disease presenting to the emergency room with a 2-week history of right lower quadrant discomfort. Physical examination reveals the presence of a small perianal fistula with drainage and right lower quadrant tenderness. Laboratory findings are significant for hemoglobin of 9.5 g dl$^{-1}$ and albumin of 2.5 g dl$^{-1}$. He undergoes a computed tomography scan that reveals thickening of the ileum extending to 30 cm with associated mesenteric inflammation and a phlegmon without an abscess. He is placed on treatment with ciprofloxacin and metronidazole and undergoes a colonoscopy that shows deep ulcerations in the ileum. Which of the following is the most effective treatment option for Kevin?

A  Start mesalamine 4.8 g daily.

B  Start azathioprine 2.5 mg kg$^{-1}$ daily.

C Start infliximab 5 mg kg$^{-1}$ every 8 weeks after a loading dose at weeks 0, 2, and 6.

D Start infliximab 5 mg kg$^{-1}$ in combination with azathioprine 2.5 mg kg$^{-1}$ daily.

4 Which of the following is the most appropriate first-line therapy in mild to moderate ileal Crohn's disease?

A Adalimumab.

B Azathioprine.

C Mesalamine.

D Budesonide.

5 Which of the following statements is *not* true about early, aggressive "top-down" therapy in patients with Crohn's disease?

A Early, aggressive therapy is associated with higher rates of mucosal healing than a step-up strategy.

B Early, aggressive therapy reduces the risk of development of penetrating complications and colorectal cancer in patients with Crohn's disease.

C Early, aggressive therapy is associated with higher rates of steroid-free remission at 1 year.

D Patients with early Crohn's disease have higher rates of response to biologic therapy than those with prolonged disease duration.

# References

1 Solem, C.A., Loftus, E.V., Jr., Tremaine, W.J., *et al.* (2005) Correlation of C-reactive protein with clinical, endoscopic, histologic, and radiographic activity in inflammatory bowel disease. *Inflammatory Bowel Diseases*, **11**(8), 707–712.

2 Rutgeerts, P., Van Assche, G., Sandborn, W.J., *et al.* (2012) Adalimumab induces and maintains mucosal healing in patients with Crohn's disease: data from the EXTEND trial. *Gastroenterology*, **142**(5), 1102–1111.e2.

3 Schnitzler, F., Fidder, H., Ferrante, M., *et al.* (2009) Mucosal healing predicts long-term outcome of maintenance therapy with infliximab in Crohn's disease. *Inflammatory Bowel Diseases*, **15**(9), 1295–1301.

4 Ananthakrishnan, A.N., Korzenik, J.R., and Hur, C. (2013) Can mucosal healing be a cost-effective endpoint for biologic therapy in Crohn's disease? A decision analysis. *Inflammatory Bowel Diseases*, **19**(1), 37–44.

5 D'Haens, G., Baert, F., van Assche, G., *et al.* (2008) Early combined immunosuppression or conventional management in patients with newly diagnosed Crohn's disease: an open randomised trial. *Lancet*, **371**(9613), 660–667.

6 Halpin, S.J. and Ford, A.C. (2012) Prevalence of symptoms meeting criteria for irritable bowel syndrome in inflammatory bowel disease: systematic review and meta-analysis. *American Journal of Gastroenterology*, **107**(10), 1474–1482.

7 Prantera, C., Lochs, H., Grimaldi, M., *et al.* (2012) Rifaximin-extended intestinal release induces remission in patients with moderately active Crohn's disease. *Gastroenterology*, **142**(3), 473–481.e4.

8 Vande Casteele, N., Gils, A., Singh, S., *et al.* (2013) Antibody response to infliximab and its impact on pharmacokinetics can be transient. *American Journal of Gastroenterology*, **108**(6), 962–971.

9 Ben-Horin, S., Waterman, M., Kopylov, U., *et al.* (2013) Addition of an immuno-modulator to infliximab therapy eliminates antidrug antibodies in serum and restores clinical response of patients with inflammatory bowel disease. *Clinical Gastroenterology and Hepatology*, **11**(4), 444–447.

10 de Silva, P.S., Nguyen, D.D., Sauk, J., *et al.* (2012) Long-term outcome of a third anti-TNF monoclonal antibody after the failure of two prior anti-TNFs in inflammatory bowel disease. *Alimentary Pharmacology & Therapeutics*, **36**(5), 459–466.

11 Allez, M., Vermeire, S., Mozziconacci, N., *et al.* (2010) The efficacy and safety of a third anti-TNF monoclonal antibody in Crohn's disease after failure of two other anti-TNF antibodies. *Alimentary Pharmacology & Therapeutics*, **31**(1), 92–101.

12 Velayos, F.S., Kahn, J.G., Sandborn, W.J., and Feagan, B.G. (2013) A test-based strategy is more cost effective than empiric dose escalation for patients with Crohn's disease who lose responsiveness to infliximab. *Clinical Gastroenterology and Hepatology*, **11**(6), 654–666.

## Answers to Questions

1  Answer: **D**. After confirming active inflammation on a colonoscopy, a test-based strategy consisting of testing drug concentrations to ensure adequate levels at trough and to assess for the presence of antidrug antibodies is more cost-effective than empiric dose escalation of infliximab [12]. Continuing infliximab without dose modification is likely to result in recurrent relapses and is not an appropriate strategy. Since Monica reports a good initial response to infliximab, this represents secondary loss of response and she is not a primary non-responder.

2  Answer: **C**. The presence of adequate trough levels and absence of antidrug antibodies suggest that the likelihood of response to a different anti-TNF biologic is low. In this scenario, switching class to an agent with a different mechanism of action is likely to be of superior benefit. Vedolizumab is an anti-$\alpha_4\beta_7$-integrin inhibitor that has established efficacy in induction and maintenance of remission in ulcerative colitis and would be an appropriate next step in this setting.

3  Answer: **D**. Kevin has several risk factors for aggressive disease course, including penetrating phenotype of disease, perianal involvement, and young age at diagnosis. As seen in the SONIC trial, a combination therapy with infliximab and azathioprine is likely to result in superior clinical and endoscopic outcomes than

using each agent as monotherapy. Consequently, this represents the best option for him. There is no evidence supporting the efficacy of mesalamine in this setting and azathioprine alone is not sufficient for induction of remission.

4  Answer: **D**. Budesonide is a systemic corticosteroid with high first-pass metabolism that has demonstrated efficacy in induction of remission in mild to moderate ileal Crohn's disease. Adalimumab is effective for inducing remission in moderate to severe Crohn's disease and is not required for those with mild disease. Aminosalicylates have not been consistently demonstrated to be effective in the treatment of Crohn's disease. Owing to a lag in its onset of action, azathioprine is not effective as first-line therapy.

5  Answer: **B**. D'Haens *et al.* performed a randomized trial comparing a conventional strategy arm (step-up) with an early aggressive therapy arm (top-down) [5]. At weeks 26 and 52, patients in the early combined arm had higher rates of steroid-free clinical remission without surgical resection compared with placebo. In addition, at 2 years, patients in the early combined treatment arm had higher rates of mucosal healing. In contrast, early aggressive therapy has not been shown to reduce rates of penetrating complications, stricture formation, or colorectal malignancy.

# 12

# Surgical Management of Inflammatory Bowel Diseases

## Clinical Take Home Messages

- Approximately 10–20% of patients with ulcerative colitis (UC) will require colectomy by 20 years after diagnosis.
- The operation of choice for UC is a total proctocolectomy with an ileal pouch–anal anastomosis (IPAA). This may be performed in one, two, or three stages.
- Pouchitis occurs in 23–50% of patients undergoing an IPAA.
- By 10 years after diagnosis, up to 60% of patients with Crohn's disease will have undergone surgery for their disease.
- Surgery in CD is not curative and eventual disease recurrence is nearly universal. Up to 80% of patients will have endoscopic recurrence within the first year after surgery and 50% may have clinical recurrence within 1 year. Factors that increase risk of recurrence include active smoking and surgery for penetrating Crohn's disease.

- The current algorithm for management of postoperative recurrence relies on tailored prophylaxis. Patients who are at low risk (i.e., those with long duration of disease or limited resection for fibrostenotic disease) can be observed clinically after the resection, and undergo active surveillance for endoscopic recurrence via colonoscopy 6–12 months after the surgery.
- Patients with one or more risk factors for recurrent disease including surgery for penetrating disease, short duration between diagnosis and first surgery, current smokers, or failure of anti-tumor necrosis factor alpha (TNF) therapy prior to first resection may benefit from initiation of anti-TNF therapy postoperatively for prevention of recurrence.

## Surgery for Ulcerative Colitis

In cohorts of patients with UC followed between 1960 and 1983, 20-year colectomy rates were as high as 68% [1]. However, cohorts with more recent diagnosis in the era of modern therapies and clinical practice have suggested reassuringly lower rates of colectomy. In the European EC-IBD cohort,

the 10-year cumulative rate of colectomy was 8.7% while a population-based study in western Hungary estimated the probability of colectomy at only 3% after 5 years of disease in those with UC diagnosed between 2002 and 2006. Corresponding analyses over the same time frame from Olmsted County, Minnesota, in the United States and the province of Manitoba in Canada identified

*Inflammatory Bowel Diseases: A Clinician's Guide*, First Edition. Ashwin N. Ananthakrishnan, Ramnik J. Xavier, and Daniel K. Podolsky.
© 2017 John Wiley & Sons Ltd. Published 2017 by John Wiley & Sons Ltd.

a 14–20% rate of colectomy 20 years after diagnosis. The decrease in colectomy rate has been less prominent among those with severe disease or early aggressive presentation than in those with moderate disease. Extent of involvement is one of the strongest predictors of colectomy, with a 3–5-fold increase in colectomy among patients with pancolitis compared with those with more limited disease.

The operation of choice for UC is a total proctocolectomy with an ileal pouch–anal anastomosis (IPAA). Total proctocolectomy is usually curative in UC and offers a particularly attractive option for patients where continued medical therapy is either ineffective or is associated with an unacceptably high risk of adverse side effects. The risk of malignancy in patients with long-standing UC may also tilt the balance towards surgery in some patients with difficult to treat disease. The option of having an ileoanal pouch and avoiding a permanent stoma is attractive to many patients when contrasted with total proctocolectomy with ileostomy, which was standard surgical practice prior to the development of the IPAA alternative. However, in addition to the operative risks, about half of patients who undergo an ileoanal pouch develop at least one episode of pouchitis. Although this frequently responds to antibiotics, recurrent pouchitis in some patients necessitates chronic antibiotic use. Furthermore, a subgroup of patients develop antibiotic-refractory pouchitis or a Crohn's-like disease of the pouch that requires immunosuppressive therapy. The pelvic dissection involved in proctectomy and creation of a J-pouch is associated with a moderate reduction in fertility, an important concern in young women. Indications for elective colectomy in UC are high-grade dysplasia or colon cancer, multifocal low-grade dysplasia, persistently active disease refractory to medical treatment, or requirement for a prolonged high dose of steroids (prednisone >15 mg per day for 6 months or longer) to maintain clinical response. Compared with elective surgery, emergency colectomy is associated with higher morbidity and mortality. Common indications for emergency surgery include toxic megacolon, fulminant colitis, free perforation, or, rarely, severe gastrointestinal hemorrhage. Even if patients with a toxic megacolon avoid surgery in the index hospitalization, they have a 50% risk of requiring surgery over the next year.

The most commonly performed surgery for UC is a total proctocolectomy with creation of an ileal pouch–anal anastomosis (IPAA) (Figure 12.1). First developed in the late 1970s by Parks and Utsunomiya, this consists of removal of the entire rectum and colon followed by creation of a J-shaped ileal pouch that functions as a reservoir. This pouch is anastomosed to the anus either with staples or with a hand-sewing technique. In a one-stage procedure, the colectomy and J-pouch creation are performed in one setting. However, this approach is associated with significant postoperative morbidity. In a two-stage procedure, the colectomy and J-pouch construction are performed with creation of a temporary ileostomy in the first stage. The second stage comprises closure of the ileostomy. A three-stage procedure is often performed when the initial surgery is for fulminant disease. In this approach, the first operation consists of a subtotal colectomy with an ileostomy. The second operation involves proctectomy with creation of the J-pouch, and the final procedure results in closure of the ileostomy. Each stage is separated in time by a few weeks. Prior to the development of the J-pouch, the most common surgery was a total proctocolectomy with a Brooke ileostomy (Figure 12.1). This remains an option for patients at high risk for incontinence or other functional problems with the pouch and those with limited mobility who would be disabled by the usual frequency of bowel movements that follows an IPAA creation. The normal expected bowel frequency with

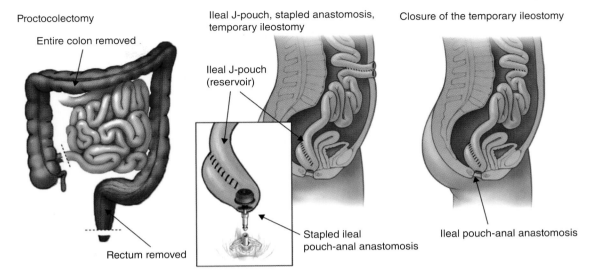

**Figure 12.1** Three-stage surgery for surgery for ulcerative colitis – total proctocolectomy with an ileal pouch–anal anastomosis (IPAA). *Source:* Adapted from Ordas *et al.* 2012 [17]. Reproduced with permission of Elsevier.

an IPAA is 5–8 bowel movements per day in addition to a nocturnal bowel movement a few times per week. Some patients require long-term antimotility agents and some develop incontinence.

Postoperative mortality after surgery for UC remains rare, between 1 and 2%. Postoperative morbidity includes wound infections, anastomotic leaks, delayed wound healing, and systemic cardiopulmonary, gastrointestinal, urinary, or infectious complications. Postoperative complications may be less frequent and the length of stay shorter in patients with laparoscopic surgery than open procedures, but high-quality comparative data with long-term follow-up are lacking.

**Pouch-related Complications in Ulcerative Colitis**

Although a total proctocolectomy with IPAA is curative for ulcerative colitis, several conditions can affect the pouch (Table 12.1) [2]. Immediate complications such as anastomotic leaks are uncommon. Pelvic sepsis,

pouch sinuses, or pouch fistulae occur in 5–20% of patients undergoing an IPAA and are more common with a one-stage procedure or in the setting of surgery for fulminant colitis. Strictures are also common after IPAA and, in a large series of 1884 patients, occurred in 11% of individuals. They are usually anastomotic or at the pouch outlet, but can occur mid-pouch or at the inlet [2]. They are treated with endoscopic dilations or exam under anesthesia with dilation in the operating room for anal strictures, but rarely require reoperation.

Pouchitis occurs in 23–50% of patients undergoing an IPAA. The incidence within 1 year of the ileostomy take down is 40% [2]. Pouchitis is almost always seen in patients undergoing surgery for UC and is very rare in patients undergoing the same procedure for treatment of familial adenomatous polyposis. The clinical presentation consists of an increase in stool frequency, urgency, incontinence, and abdominal cramping or pelvic discomfort. In some patients, it may be due to superimposed infection such as

**Table 12.1** Classification of ileal pouch disorders and associated complications.

| | |
|---|---|
| Surgical and mechanical | Anastomotic leaks |
| | Pelvic sepsis and abscess |
| | Pouch sinuses |
| | Pouch fistulae |
| | Strictures |
| | Afferent limb syndrome and efferent limb syndrome |
| | Infertility and sexual dysfunction |
| | Portal vein thrombi |
| | Pouch prolapse, twisted pouch bleeding, sphincter injury or dysfunction |
| Inflammatory and infectious | Pouchitis |
| | Cuffitis |
| | CD of the pouch |
| | Proximal small-bowel bacterial overgrowth |
| | Inflammatory polyps |
| Functional | Irritable pouch syndrome |
| | Anismus |
| | Pseudo-obstruction |
| Dysplastic and neoplastic | Dysplasia or cancer of the pouch |
| | Dysplasia or cancer of the anal transitional zone |
| Systemic and metabolic | Anemia |
| | Bone loss |
| | Vitamin $B_{12}$ deficiency |

*Source:* Shen *et al.* 2008 [2]. Reproduced with permission of Elsevier.

*Clostridium difficile* infection [3]. Both ciprofloxacin and metronidazole are good first-line agents for the treatment of pouchitis (Figure 12.2). Some patients require just a single 2-week course of antibiotics but others may need multiple courses and a subset of patients may be dependent on chronic antibiotic therapy. Chronic antibiotic-refractory pouchitis (failure to respond to a 4-week course of antibiotics) may require combination of antibiotics, initiation of immunomodulator or biologic therapy or rarely, removal of the pouch.

Cuffitis refers to inflammation of the rectal cuff in patients in whom the anastomosis is made without mucosectomy. In essence, it represents continuation of UC in the residual rectal mucosa. Its symptoms may be indistinguishable from pouchitis. It is usually treated with topical 5-aminosalicylates or topic corticosteroids. Crohn's disease (CD) of the pouch occurs in 2–10% of patients who undergo an IPAA and is more common in those with preoperative diagnosis of indeterminate colitis. The behavior of this CD-like pouch inflammation ranges from inflammatory to penetrating disease as for *de novo* CD. Endoscopic features suggestive of CD of the pouch include ulcerations in the afferent limb, stricture at the pouch inlet, and strictures or ulcers at other parts of the small bowel. The management of CD of the pouch is similar to that of luminal CD. Rarely, patients with an ileoanal pouch

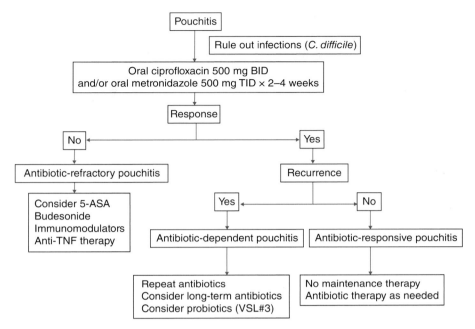

**Figure 12.2** Algorithm for management of pouchitis. Anti-TNF, monoclonal antibodies to tumor necrosis factor alpha; 5-ASA, 5-aminosalicylates.

develop cancer in the anal transition zone, particularly in patients who have the stapled anastomosis without mucosectomy. Although there is controversy in the literature about the need for routine surveillance in such individuals, patients who undergo colectomy for dysplasia or cancer are at an increased risk for colon cancer in the anal transition zone and should undergo annual or biannual surveillance colonoscopies.

## Surgery for Crohn's Disease

Within 10 years after diagnosis of CD, up to 60% of patients will have undergone surgery for their disease. Unlike UC, surgery in CD is not curative as disease recurrence is the norm. Up to 80% of patients have endoscopic recurrence within the first year after surgery and 50% have clinical recurrence within 1 year. The cumulative risk of recurrence requiring reoperation is 33–58% 10

years after the initial surgery. The most common indications for intestinal surgery in CD are failure of medical management and development of penetrating or stricturing complications such as an ileocecal abscess, internal fistulae, or small-bowel strictures with repeated episodes of bowel obstruction from fibrostenosis. Risk factors for repeat surgery include current smoking and initial surgery for small-bowel penetrating disease. The principles of surgery for CD are distinct from UC owing to risk of recurrence and likelihood of eventual repeat surgery. Thus, an important concept in the management of CD disease surgically is limited resection or bowel-preserving techniques such as strictureplasty. A randomized controlled trial (RCT) comparing limited and extended resection found no benefit in preventing recurrence through the adoption of wide margins [4].

The most common surgery performed in patients with ileocolonic CD is ileocecal resection with primary anastomosis of the neoterminal ileum to the ascending colon. This can be accomplished either as open surgery or laparoscopically. In a systematic review of laparoscopic versus open surgery for small-bowel CD, laparoscopic resection was associated with reduced rates of wound infection and non-disease-related complications but was not statistically superior to open surgery. There was no difference in long-term reoperation rates between laparoscopic and open surgery [5], suggesting that where expertise is available, laparoscopic surgery is a suitable option for patients.

In patients with small-bowel stricture, bowel-sparing techniques, most commonly strictureplasty, are increasingly used. A strictureplasty consists in making a longitudinal incision on the stricture with subsequent transverse closure that increases the luminal diameter. A strictureplasty preserves the small bowel and reduces the risk of development of short-bowel syndrome. Patients who have less than 100–200 cm of bowel are at risk for malabsorption and dependence on total parenteral nutrition. Strictureplasties are traditionally used for short fibrotic stricture not associated with active disease, although reports have demonstrated that it can be safely and effectively performed even in the setting of active inflammation or for longer strictures [6]. Strictureplasties are most effective in jejunal or ileal disease. The 5-year recurrence rate after strictureplasty was 28% in a large meta-analysis and, in a majority of patients, recurrence occurred at a non-strictureplasty site [7]. Strictureplasty has also been described as a safe and effective option for the management of gastroduodenal CD [8, 9]. Rare cases of small intestinal adenocarcinoma have been reported at the site of strictureplasty [10, 11]. Distal ileal strictures may be amenable to endoscopic balloon dilatation as an alternative.

The rate of surgical resection is lower in patients with colonic CD. The operations commonly performed in such patients included either a segmental colectomy (for example, for a colonic stricture) or a subtotal colectomy for medically refractory disease with similar recurrence-free survival between the two groups [12, 13]. As rectal involvement is infrequent or mild in patients with CD, subtotal colectomy with an ileorectal anastomosis may be a reasonable option in patients with a normal rectum. For patients with rectal disease, the procedure of choice is total proctocolectomy with Brooke ileostomy. Ileoanal pouch surgeries have been reported in some patients with colonic CD but may be associated with higher rates of pouch failure [14]. The management of perianal and fistulizing CD is addressed in Chapter 13.

## Prophylaxis for Prevention of Postoperative Recurrence in Crohn's Disease

As endoscopic recurrence is seen in nearly 80% of patients at 1 year, with clinical recurrence in over 50%, the identification of subgroups at high risk of recurrence and initiation of appropriate therapy to prevent recurrence are important. Factors that increase risk of recurrence include active smoking and surgery for penetrating CD, and other less well-established risk factors include extent of bowel resection, presence of granulomas, histologic activity at the margin, and type of anastomosis. Several studies have been conducted to evaluate the efficacy of various therapies in the prevention of postoperative recurrence.

Aminosalicylates have a weak effect in recurrence prevention. In a meta-analysis, clinical recurrence at 12 months was lower in a group treatment with mesalamine compared with placebo (relative risk 0.76, 95% confidence interval 0.62–0.94), although none of the individual trials met statistical significance [15]. Mesalamine also reduced endoscopic recurrence and

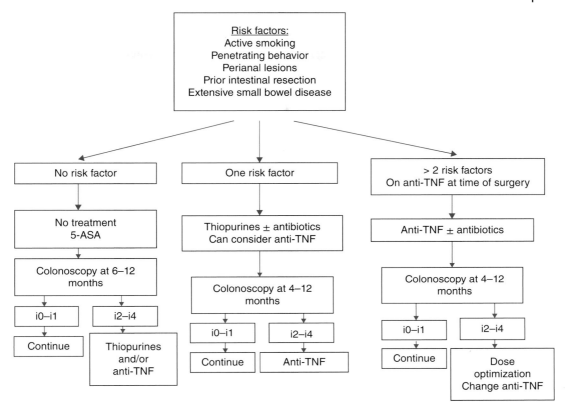

**Figure 12.3** Algorithm for postoperative prophylaxis to prevent recurrence in Crohn's disease. Anti-TNF, monoclonal antibodies to tumor necrosis factor alpha; 5-ASA, 5-aminosalicylates; i0–i4, Rutgeerts postoperative classification.

severe endoscopic recurrence at 12 months. Substantial data confirm the efficacy of antibiotics, particularly nitroimidazoles. In RCTs, both metronidazole and ornidazole were effective in preventing clinical and endoscopic recurrence when administered for 3 months and 1 year, respectively, but are poorly tolerated. Four trials of azathioprine demonstrated lower rates of clinical and endoscopic recurrence with azathioprine compared with 5-ASA or placebo. A small proof of concept study by Regueiro *et al.* [16] yielded the most promising data in support of prevention of postoperative recurrence. They randomized 24 patients to either infliximab or placebo. At the end of 1 year, infliximab was associated with a 9%

rate of endoscopic recurrence compared with 85% with placebo. The clinical remission rates were 80% with infliximab compared with 54% with placebo. Larger trials are under way to establish the benefit of prophylactic biologics.

The current algorithm for management of postoperative recurrence prophylaxis relies on tailored prophylaxis (Figure 12.3). Patients at low risk – those with long duration of disease or limited resection for fibrostenotic disease – may be observed clinically after the resection. Since endoscopic recurrence universally precedes clinical recurrence and severity of endoscopic recurrence is an important prognostic marker, colonoscopy should be performed 6–12 months after the resection even in the absence of symptoms to determine the need to step up therapy if based on significant endoscopic recurrence. Patients with one or more risk factors for recurrent disease, such as surgery for penetrating disease, short duration between diagnosis and first surgery, current smokers, or failure of anti-TNF therapy prior to first resection, may benefit from initiation of anti-TNF therapy postoperatively for prevention of recurrence. The efficacy of biologics appears to be superior when administered early after surgery compared with use as treatment for recurrent disease.

## Case Studies and Multiple Choice Questions

1  Jacob had a 5-year history of ileal Crohn's disease which was refractory to azathioprine and infliximab. He then underwent a laparoscopic ileocecal resection with a side-to-side anastomosis and was placed on adalimumab for prevention of postoperative recurrence of Crohn's disease. A colonoscopy was performed 6 months after the surgery and revealed three apthae at the anastomosis. Which of the following statements is accurate?

A  This is classified as i0 according to the Rutgeerts classification and does not require escalation of therapy.

B  This is classified as i1 according to the Rutgeerts classification and does not require escalation of therapy.

C  This is classified as i2 according to the Rutgeerts classification and should be managed by addition of metronidazole.

D  This is classified as i3 according to the Rutgeerts classification and would suggest a need for increasing the dose of adalimumab to weekly administration.

2  Which of the following agents is associated with reduced risk of recurrence of Crohn's disease following ileocecal resection?

A  Ciprofloxacin.
B  Metronidazole.
C  Rifaximin.
D  Budesonide.

3  Which of the following statements is *not* true about pouchitis after ileal pouch–anal anastomosis surgery?

A  The first line-treatment for acute pouchitis is ciprofloxacin and metronidazole.

B  The first-line treatment for pouchitis is systemic corticosteroid therapy.

C  Pouchitis can occur in up to 50% of patients who undergo J-pouch surgery.

D  Most patients with pouchitis do not require immunosuppressive therapy.

# References

1 Farmer, R.G., Easley, K.A., and Rankin, G.B. (1993) Clinical patterns, natural history, and progression of ulcerative colitis. A long-term follow-up of 1116 patients. *Digestive Diseases and Sciences*, **38**(6), 1137–1146.

2 Shen, B., Remzi, F.H., Lavery, I.C., *et al.* (2008) A proposed classification of ileal pouch disorders and associated complications after restorative proctocolectomy. *Clinical Gastroenterology and Hepatology*, **6**(2), 145–158; quiz, 24.

3 Shen, B., Jiang, Z.-D., Fazio, V.W., *et al.* (2008) *Clostridium difficile* infection in patients with ileal pouch-anal anastomosis. *Clinical Gastroenterology and Hepatolog*, **6**(7), 782–788.

4 Sales, D.J. and Kirsner, J.B. (1983) The prognosis of inflammatory bowel disease. *Archives of Internal Medicine*, **143**(2), 294–299.

5 Dasari, B.V., McKay, D., and Gardiner, K. (2011) Laparoscopic versus open surgery for small bowel Crohn's disease. *Cochrane Database of Systematic Reviews*, (**1**), CD006956.

6 Shatari, T., Clark, M.A., Yamamoto, T., *et al.* (2004) Long strictureplasty is as safe and effective as short strictureplasty in small-bowel Crohn's disease. *Colorectal Disease*, **6**(6), 438–441.

7 Yamamoto, T., Fazio, V.W., and Tekkis, P.P. (2007) Safety and efficacy of strictureplasty for Crohn's disease: a systematic review and meta-analysis. *Diseases of the Colon and Rectum*, **50**(11), 1968–1986.

8 Tonelli, F., Alemanno, G., Bellucci, F., *et al.* (2013) Symptomatic duodenal Crohn's disease: is strictureplasty the right choice? *Journal of Crohn's & Colitis*, **7**(10), 791–796.

9 Worsey, M.J., Hull, T., Ryland, L., and Fazio, V. (1999) Strictureplasty is an effective option in the operative management of duodenal Crohn's disease. *Diseases of the Colon and Rectum*, **42**(5), 596–600.

10 Menon, A.M., Mirza, A.H., Moolla, S., and Morton, D.G. (2007) Adenocarcinoma of the small bowel arising from a previous strictureplasty for Crohn's disease: report of a case. *Diseases of the Colon and Rectum*, **50**(2), 257–259.

11 Partridge, S.K. and Hodin, R.A. (2004) Small bowel adenocarcinoma at a strictureplasty site in a patient with Crohn's disease: report of a case. *Diseases of the Colon and Rectum*, **47**(5), 778–781.

12 Kiran, R.P., Nisar, P.J., Church, J.M., and Fazio, V.W. (2011) The role of primary surgical procedure in maintaining intestinal continuity for patients with Crohn's colitis. *Annals of Surgery*, **253**(6), 1130–1135.

13 Fichera, A., McCormack, R., Rubin, M.A., *et al.* (2005) Long-term outcome of surgically treated Crohn's colitis: a

prospective study. *Diseases of the Colon and Rectum*, **48**(5), 963–969.

14 Le, Q., Melmed, G., Dubinsky, M., *et al.* (2013) Surgical outcome of ileal pouch–anal anastomosis when used intentionally for well-defined Crohn's disease. *Inflammatory Bowel Diseases*, **19**(1), 30–36.

15 Doherty, G., Bennett, G., Patil, S., *et al.* (2009) Interventions for prevention of post-operative recurrence of Crohn's disease. *Cochrane Database of Systematic Reviews*, (**4**), CD006873.

16 Regueiro, M., Schraut, W., Baidoo, L., *et al.* (2009) Infliximab prevents Crohn's disease recurrence after ileal resection. *Gastroenterology*, **136**(2), 441–450.e1; quiz, 716.

17 Ordas, I., Eckmann, L., Talamini, M., *et al.* (2012) Ulcerative colitis. *Lancet*, **380**(9853), 1606–1619.

## Recommended Reading

Nguyen, G.C., Loftus, E.V., Hirano, I., *et al.* (2017) American Gastroenterological Association Institute guideline on the management of Crohn's Disease after surgical resection. *American Journal of Gastroenterology*, **152**(1), 271–275.

Regueiro, M., Velayos, F., Greer, J.B., *et al.* (2017) American Gastroenterological Association Institute guideline on the management of Crohn's Disease after surgical resection. *American Journal of Gastroenterology*, **152**(1), 277–295.

## Answers to Questions

1   Answer: **B**. The presence of fewer than five aphthous ulcers in the neoterminal ileum is classified as i1 according to the Rutgeerts classification and is associated with low risk of progression or need for recurrent surgery. It would be reasonable to continue Jacob on the adalimumab without escalation in therapy and plan repeat endoscopic surveillance in 1 year. Although there are data supporting the role of metronidazole in prevention of postoperative recurrence, there are no RCT data supporting its efficacy in treating recurrent Crohn's disease.

2   Answer: **B**. In RCTs, both metronidazole and ornidazole were effective in prevent-ing clinical and endoscopic recurrence when administered for 3 months and 1 year, respectively. There are no data sup-porting a benefit from use of the other agents for prevention of recurrence of Crohn's disease.

3   Answer: **B**. Pouchitis, which occurs in 50% of patients following a J-pouch sur-gery, typically responds to antibiotic therapy and not systemic corticoster-oids. Only a small subset of patients with pouchitis develop chronic, antibiotic-refractory symptoms and require initia-tion of immunosuppressive therapy.

# 13

# Complications of Inflammatory Bowel Diseases

## Clinical Take Home Messages

- A new colonic stricture in patients with established ulcerative colitis (UC), particularly in those with underlying primary sclerosing cholangitis (PSC) or longstanding disease, should raise suspicion for underlying malignancy, Crohn's disease (CD), or other etiologies such as ischemic or diverticular stricture.
- There has been a recent increase in the incidence of *Clostridium difficile* infection among patients with inflammatory bowel disease (IBD). This infection is associated with increased risk for morbidity and mortality. All patients with symptomatic disease flares, ambulatory or hospitalized, should be tested for *C. difficile*.
- Reactivation of cytomegalovirus (CMV) in the colon, termed CMV colitis, can complicate the course of up to one-third of patients with steroid-refractory disease and is diagnosed by immunohistochemistry, polymerase chain reaction, or culture from colonic biopsies of involved areas.
- Both UC and CD are associated with an increased risk for colorectal cancer. Diagnosis at a younger age, extensive disease, longer duration of disease, coexisting PSC, and severity of inflammation are associated with increased risk for colorectal neoplasia.
- Dysplasia may be unifocal or multifocal, and can be invisible endoscopically (flat dysplasia) or visible as endoscopically raised lesions. Endoscopically visible dysplasia may be amenable to resection in the case of small polypoid lesions. In contrast, unifocal or multifocal high-grade flat dysplasia is usually managed with colectomy.
- Fibrostenosis or strictures develop in 18% of patients with CD by 20 years after diagnosis, most commonly in the terminal ileum. Endoscopic balloon dilation is effective for short strictures involving the ileum or for anastomotic strictures, but definitive treatment usually requires surgical resection or, where possible, bowel-conserving procedures such as strictureplasty.
- Perianal or enterocutaneous fistulae occur in 35% of patients with CD. Anti-tumor necrosis factor biologics are effective in the treatment of perianal CD. Rectovaginal or enterovesical fistulae often have poor response to medical treatment and frequently require surgical intervention.
- Severe Ulcerative Colitis can lead to Toxic Megacolon and/or perforation, a dire complication usually requiring emergent colectomy.

*Inflammatory Bowel Diseases: A Clinician's Guide*, First Edition. Ashwin N. Ananthakrishnan, Ramnik J. Xavier, and Daniel K. Podolsky.
© 2017 John Wiley & Sons Ltd. Published 2017 by John Wiley & Sons Ltd.

# Complications of Ulcerative Colitis

### Toxic Megacolon and Perforation

Toxic megacolon is a feared complication of acute severe colitis. It is defined clinically by dilation of the colonic lumen to 6 cm or greater, often accompanied by abdominal pain, fever, tachycardia, hypotension, electrolyte abnormalities, and/or altered mental status. In patients with acute severe colitis, sudden cessation of bowel movements or abdominal distension should trigger suspicion for this complication. The abdomen will appear distended and tympanitic on percussion, and bowel sounds are absent. This complication is usually evident on a plain abdominal film (Figure 13.1). Immediate management consists of stopping potential triggers such as narcotics and anticholinergics and also correction of contributing electrolyte abnormalities. Early surgical consultation is critical. Decompression may be attempted by rolling the patient on to the right-lateral or prone position, and placement of a nasogastric and rectal tube. Intravenous steroids and antibiotics, if not already begun, should be initiated and serial abdominal X-rays obtained every 6–12 h for signs of progressive dilation or extraluminal free air indicating perforation. Endoscopic evaluation should be avoided owing to risk of perforation. Toxic megacolon is associated with high rates of mortality and frequently necessitates urgent colectomy.

Abrupt onset of fever and peritoneal signs may indicate a free perforation, which is a rare complication of severe colitis. It can occur even in the absence of toxic megacolon and is also associated with high mortality in the absence of urgent surgery. The diagnosis is established on physical examination and cross-sectional imaging with a computed tomography (CT) scan. Broad-spectrum antibiotics should immediately be initiated along with restoration of fluid electrolyte balance and correction of associated comorbidities such as anemia. Endoscopic evaluation or barium studies should be avoided in suspected free perforation.

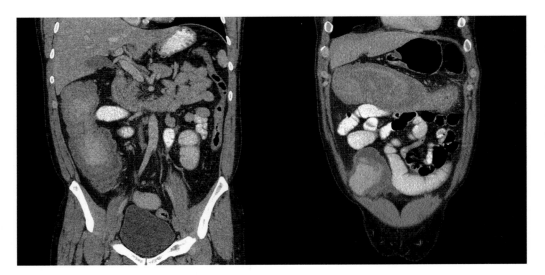

Figure 13.1 Computed tomography images of toxic megacolon in a patient with severe ulcerative colitis.

## Colonic Strictures

Because the inflammation is limited to the submucosa and mucosa in ulcerative colitis (UC), colonic strictures as a consequence of long-standing inflammation are uncommon compared with Crohn's disease (CD). A new colonic stricture, particularly in patients with underlying primary sclerosing cholangitis (PSC) or longstanding disease, should raise suspicion for underlying malignancy, CD, or other etiologies such as ischemic or diverticular stricture. Until proven otherwise, a stricture in UC should be presumed to be malignant. Multiple biopsies of both the stricture and the surrounding mucosa should be obtained. In some cases, cross-sectional imaging is useful to establish a diagnosis. In cases where high suspicion for a malignancy underlying the stricture remains, surgery is the appropriate treatment strategy both to provide a diagnosis and to treat the consequences of the stricture. If strictures cannot be bypassed endoscopically, thus precluding surveillance of the proximal colon in patients with longstanding disease, surgical resection should be considered.

## *Clostridium difficile* and Cytomegalovirus Colitis

There has been a recent increase in the incidence of *Clostridium difficile* infection among patients with IBD. In some series, as many as half of patients with acute severe colitis have been found to have superimposed *C. difficile* infection [1]. *C. difficile* infection in patients with UC is associated with both excess morbidity and mortality. In a large study of hospitalized patients, occurrence of *C. difficile* infection was associated with a sixfold greater mortality [2]. Other studies have demonstrated a greater need for therapy escalation and a higher rate of colectomy in those with *C. difficile* [3]. It is important to have a high index of suspicion for *C. difficile* infection in patients with UC as traditional risk factors such as prior healthcare exposure or antibiotic use occur less frequently in this cohort than in those who develop *C. difficile* infection in the absence of underlying IBD. Use of systemic steroid, ongoing immunosuppression, and extent of colitis are risk factors for *C. difficile* in patients with IBD. Clinically, *C. difficile* infection may be indistinguishable from a UC colitis flare. The diagnosis is established by demonstration of the toxin in stool through either enzyme-linked immunosorbent assay (ELISA) or polymerase chain reaction (PCR). Pseudomembranes, a classical feature of *C. difficile* colitis, are infrequent in patients with IBD, and their absence should not rule out this diagnosis. Metronidazole is a treatment option for very mild disease. However, for those with more severe disease, oral vancomycin may be the appropriate initial treatment given the higher success rates in those with severe *C. difficile* infection.

Primary cytomegalovirus (CMV) infection is uncommon in patients with IBD. However, reactivation of CMV in the colon, termed CMV colitis, is relatively common, particularly in those receiving corticosteroid or other immunosuppressive agents. It complicates up to one-third of patients with steroid-refractory disease [4, 5]. The diagnosis is established by obtaining a biopsy from the ulcer base on flexible sigmoidoscopy and demonstrating viral inclusions on histology or immunohistochemistry, with the latter being more sensitive. PCR testing and rapid viral culture ("shell vial culture") are also available as relatively rapid tests to establish a diagnosis of CMV colitis. Serologic testing for CMV antibodies, antigenemia, or viral copies in the circulation by PCR are usually not helpful in differentiating CMV infection from CMV disease and have poor sensitivity and specificity for establishing a diagnosis of latent CMV colitis. There is debate in the literature on whether CMV is truly pathogenic in this setting or is an "innocent bystander." However, in patients refractory to corticosteroids or biologics, initiation of intravenous ganciclovir for 3–5 days followed by a 14–21-day course of oral valganciclovir is associated with good rates of improvement.

### Colorectal Dysplasia and Cancer

#### Magnitude and Risk Factors

Both UC and CD are associated with an increased risk for colorectal cancer. Estimates of the magnitude of this risk have varied. In the initial studies on the incidence of colorectal cancer, summarized in a meta-analysis by Eaden *et al.* [6], the risk was estimated to be 2% after 10 years, 8% after 20 years, and 18% after 30 years of disease. However, more recent analyses have suggested that the risk is lower. In a large, prospective observational cohort in France that included 19 486 patients with IBD, 37 developed colorectal cancer and 20 developed high-grade dysplasia, yielding a standardized incidence ratio of 2 for all patients with IBD and 7 for patients with longstanding colitis [7]. This temporal decline in cancer risk was also observed in a Scandinavian study in which the relative risk for colorectal cancer decreased from 1.34 in 1979–1988 to 0.57 in more recent cohorts with only patients with extensive pancolitis, young age at diagnosis, or male gender being at increased risk [8, 9]. Potential factors contributing towards this secular decrease include more effective medical therapy, more frequent enrollment in colorectal cancer surveillance programs, and higher rates of proctocolectomy in patients with dysplasia or medical treatment failures. Patients with ulcerative proctitis are not at increased risk for colorectal cancer and do not merit more frequent surveillance examinations. Patients with CD with extensive colitis involving more than one-third of their colon are at the same risk for colorectal cancer as those with UC [10].

There are several established risk factors for colorectal neoplasia in patients with IBD (Table 13.1). Diagnosis at a younger age,

**Table 13.1** Risk factors for colorectal neoplasia in patients with inflammatory bowel disease.

| Duration of disease |
| --- |
| Extent of involvement |
| Coexisting primary sclerosing cholangitis |
| Multiple inflammatory pseudopolyps |
| Colonic strictures |
| Family history of colorectal cancer |
| Severity of inflammation |
| Young age at diagnosis |

extensive disease, and longer duration of disease are all associated with increased risk for colorectal neoplasia. Coexisting PSC is associated with a substantial increase in risk for colorectal cancer. Severity of and histologic or elevated serum inflammatory markers are also associated with an increased risk for colorectal cancer or dysplasia [11, 12]. Other risk factors for colorectal cancer in IBD include family history of colon cancer, colonic strictures, a shortened colon, and multiple post-inflammatory pseudopolyps [13]. In contrast, undergoing regular surveillance examinations is associated with decreased risk for colorectal cancer and lower mortality following a diagnosis of colon cancer.

The molecular basis of colitis-associated cancer differs from that of sporadic colon cancer. In sporadic cancer, the loss of function of the adenomatous polyposis coli (*APC*) gene is an early event and *p53* mutations occur late in the adenoma–carcinoma cycle. In contrast, in IBD-associated colon cancers, *p53* mutations occur early and loss of *APC* is a late event. Colon cancer developing in the context of IBD tends to be multicentric, and more likely to occur in flat mucosa, appearing as flat, plaque-like lesions that may be less distinctly visualized than in the general population.

## Surveillance for Dysplasia and Cancer

Dysplasia, manifested histologically by nuclear stratification, nuclear and cellular polymorphism, and lack of nuclear polarity, represents neoplastic transformation in the epithelium without penetration of the lamina propria [13]. It is stratified into low- and high-grade dysplasia (LGD and HGD, respectively), but in some cases may be indeterminate and difficult to distinguish from inflammation-related changes. Although colon cancer can develop without preceding dysplasia, the high frequency of preceding dysplasia (75–90%) in patients who eventually develop colon cancer led to recommendations for routine surveillance. Both the American Gastroenterological Association and British Society of Gastroenterology recommend surveillance colonoscopies beginning at 8–10 years after symptoms. Each surveillance exam should entail high-quality visualization of the colon mucosa with random four-quadrant biopsies obtained every 10 cm in the colon, for a total of at least 33 biopsies. In addition, visible or polypoid lesions should be biopsied separately. Repeat examinations should be carried out every 1–3 years after the initial screening exam in patients without primary PSC and annually in those with PSC. Other than patients with sclerosing cholangitis, guidelines do not offer firm recommendations on modifying screening intervals based on other risk factors. Most surveillance programs utilize standard or high-definition white light endoscopy. However, several studies have demonstrated greater sensitivity with chromoendoscopy. In a study by Rutter *et al.*, chromoendoscopy found seven dysplastic lesions out of 157 targeted biopsies compared with no dysplasia in 2904 non-targeted biopsies [14]. Thus, chromoendoscopy with targeted biopsies is also an accepted screening strategy.

## Management of Dysplasia

Key principles defining the management of dysplasia in patients with IBD are the higher likelihood of progression to colorectal cancer and the significant frequency of malignancy in colons resected for dysplasia. Dysplasia can be unifocal or multifocal, and may be invisible endoscopically (flat dysplasia) or visible as endoscopically raised lesions. Endoscopically visible dysplasia may be amenable to resection in the case of small polypoid lesions. Endomucosal resection may be useful for larger but well-circumscribed lesions, although flat endoscopically visible dysplasic lesions may be associated with a higher rate of colon cancer (38–83% in retrospective cohorts) [13].

The management of dysplasia depends on both the degree and type of dysplasia. Adenoma-like lesions that are amenable to endoscopic polypectomy, regardless of the degree of dysplasia, and that have no dysplasia in the surrounding mucosa or elsewhere in the colon, can be managed conservatively with no need for accelerated surveillance. The rate of subsequent dysplasia or cancer in this setting is low [13]. In contrast, unifocal or multifocal high-grade flat dysplasia is usually managed with colectomy as synchronous colon cancer is present in 42–67% of cases and these patients otherwise remain at high risk for cancer on follow-up. In contrast, management of LGD is challenging owing to the varying rates of progression (0–54%) reported in the literature. In a small study by Ullman *et al.*, one-third of patients with LGD progressed to advanced lesions at 5 years [15]; Zisman *et al.* identified only a 19% rate of progression at 4 years [16] and Pekow *et al.* identified only a 4.3 per 100 person-years risk of progression [17]. In contrast, in an earlier series of 46 patients who underwent colectomy for flat low-grade dysplasia as the most advanced lesion, 24% had unexpected advanced neoplasia, yielding a rate of progression of 53% at 5 years [18]. Multifocal LGD, after confirmation by a second pathologist, is usually a basis to recommend total proctocolectomy. Although surgery remains an acceptable treatment option for unifocal LGD, such lesions can be managed by surveillance examinations with a repeat colonoscopy in 3–6 months, and subsequently every 6 months until there are at least two surveillance examinations with no dysplasia detected. Chromoendoscopy is a particularly attractive option in such patients.

### Chemoprevention

There are limited prospective data assessing the efficacy of chemoprevention in IBD. Initial case–control [19] and cohort studies [20] summarized in a meta-analysis [21] suggested a protective effect of aminosalicylates on colorectal cancer risk in IBD. However, more recent population-based studies failed to find this protective effect [22, 23]. An earlier study also suggested that ursodeoxycholic acid (UDCA), used in patients with UC and PSC, was associated with a lower risk for colon cancer (relative risk 0.26, 95% confidence interval 0.06–0.92) [24, 25]. In contrast, in a more recent study, higher doses of UDCA of 28–30 mg kg$^{-1}$

were associated with an increased risk for colorectal neoplasia in UC [26]. Hence routine use of either aminosalicylates or UDCA as chemoprevention does not appear warranted.

## Complications of Crohn's Disease

### Fibrostenosis and Strictures

Fibrostenosis or strictures develop in 18% of patients with CD within 20 years following diagnosis. The most common site of involvement is the terminal ileum (Figure 13.2). Patients usually present with abdominal pain, reduction in their frequency of bowel movements, or abdominal distension typically 30–90 min following food intake. Strictures may be inflammatory and respond to escalation of their medical treatment. Obstruction due to strictures that are primarily fibrotic in nature usually does not respond to systemic treatment escalation and often requires endoscopic or surgical therapy. All patients with significant strictures should be placed on a low-residue diet and advised to avoid intake of materials that may be poorly

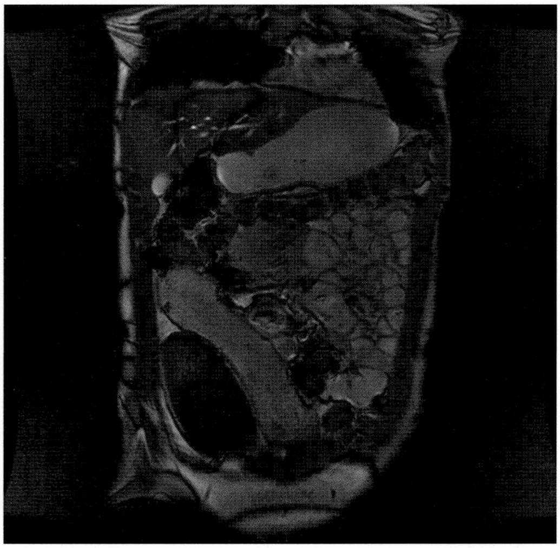

Figure 13.2 Magnetic resonance enterography image of terminal ileal stricture and high-grade small-bowel obstruction in a patient with Crohn's disease.

digested, including raw fruits, vegetables, nuts, seeds, and corn. The definitive treatment for significant fibrostenotic strictures is surgery, either resection or, where possible, bowel-conserving procedures such as strictureplasty. Endoscopic balloon dilation is effective for short strictures involving the ileum or for anastomotic strictures [27]. There is limited literature supporting endoscopic dilation of primary Crohn's strictures. Intra-lesional steroids [28] and infliximab [29] injections have shown short-term success but limited data exist to support them as durable interventions.

### Abscesses

Owing to the transmural nature of inflammation in CD, abscesses occur at some point in over half of people with the disease. These abscesses may be intra-abdominal, most commonly adjacent to the ileum. Back pain or pain radiating down the thigh may indicate a psoas abscess. Patients with an intra-abdominal abscess may present with abdominal pain alone or in conjunction with

systemic features such as fevers or chills. In patients who are on immunosuppressive therapy, particularly corticosteroids, systemic features can be masked. If the abscess cavity is sealed off with an inflammatory phlegmon, systemic features or peritoneal findings may not be apparent. Laboratory evaluation reveals an elevated white blood cell count and markedly elevated measures of inflammation. The diagnosis of an abscess requires an abdominal–pelvic CT scan with both oral and intravenous contrast. Magnetic resonance imaging (MRI) may also be useful to image an abscess, although CT scanning has the advantage that guided drainage procedures may be performed.

The first step in the management of an intra-abdominal abscess is drainage, often performed with ultrasound or CT guidance (Figure 13.3). Drains may need to be left in place for a few weeks with periodic irrigation of the abscess cavity, sometimes requiring lysis of adhesions that result in loculated collections. Antibiotics are used for 2–4 weeks, ciprofloxacin and metronidazole being good initial choices. Culture of

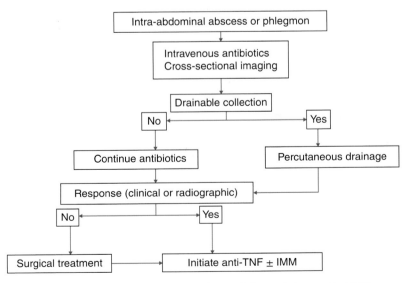

**Figure 13.3** Algorithm for management of intra-abdominal abscess. Anti-TNF, monoclonal antibodies to tumor necrosis factor alpha; IMM, immunomodulator.

organisms from the abscess cavity or blood can guide further tailoring of the antibiotic regimen. Corticosteroid use or escalation of biologic therapy should be avoided in the setting of an undrained abscess, although patients already on such therapies may need to have them continued.

Traditionally, early surgical intervention with resection of the diseased segment was the modality of choice for treatment of intra-abdominal abscesses. However, emerging data suggest that early interventional drainage, antibiotics, and continued medical therapy may delay or avoid the need for surgery. In a series of 95 patients with an abdominal abscess, the median duration of hospitalization was 15.5 days in patients who underwent surgery compared with 5 days in those who did not [30]. The probability of abscess recurrence was similar in the two groups (31% vs. 20%) and initiation of anti-tumor necrosis factor (TNF) therapy was associated with reduced risk of abscess recurrence. Only 12 out of 55 patients who were initially treated non-surgically eventually required an operation for management of their disease. This, along with other emerging literature, indicates that percutaneous drainage, antibiotics, and subsequent effective medical therapy for CD may allow surgery to be avoided in a subset of patients [30]. Patients with an inflammatory phlegmon may benefit from antibiotics and concomitant steroids to treat the associated luminal inflammation. Such patients often need surgery, but a subset of patients can be safely and effectively managed with antibiotics and anti-TNF therapy. In a series of 13 such patients, only two eventually required surgery, both more than 1 year after initiating anti-TNF treatment [31].

### Fistulizing Crohn's Disease

Perianal or enterocutaneous fistulae occur in 35% of patients with CD [32]. In a population-based study in Olmsted County, Minnesota, the cumulative risk of any fistula 10 and 20 years after diagnosis was 33% and 50%, respectively. Most of the fistulae were perianal (51%), a small proportion were rectovaginal (9%), and the remainder were internal or enterocutaneous [32]. Most patients who had fistulae required surgery and one-third developed recurrence of the fistulae [32]. Fistulae develop either as a result of transmural inflammation of the bowel, leading to penetration into adjacent organs or loops of bowel, or secondary to a distal stricture, leading to dilation of the proximal segment of the bowel and subsequent fistula formation. Some fistulae may be asymptomatic (e.g., enteroenteric fistulae) or cause symptoms depending on the location of involvement. Perianal fistulae often present as pain from the fistula, formation of an abscess, or drainage from the perianal region. Gastrocolonic or enterosigmoid fistulae may present as diarrhea. Enterovesicular fistulae present as recurrent urinary tract infection, polymicrobial urinary infections, pneumaturia, or fecaluria. Rectovaginal fistulae present as drainage of stool or mucous through the vagina.

Perianal fistulae are classified by their relationship to the internal and external anal sphincter, and their relationship in the intersphincteric plane, which has important implications for treatment. They can be classified as (1) intersphincteric, (2) transsphincteric, (3) suprasphincteric, (4) extrasphincteric, and (5) superficial, depending on their relationship to the external anal sphincter (Figure 13.4). The superficial fistula is external to both the internal and external anal sphincter complexes; an intersphincteric fistula tracks between the internal and external sphincter complexes; the suprasphincteric fistula enters the rectum over the top of the puborectalis muscle; and the trans-sphincteric fistula tracks through the external anal sphincter. An alternative system of classification subgroups the fistulae as either simple or complex. Simple

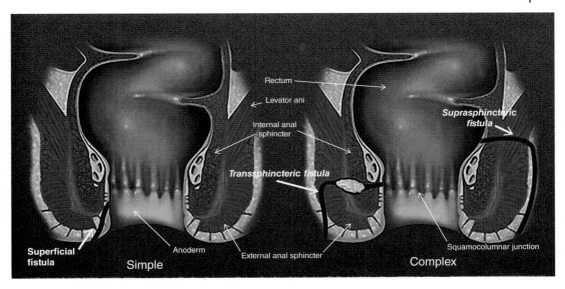

**Figure 13.4** Types of perianal fistulae in Crohn's disease. *Source:* Adapted from Schwartz and Maltz 2009 [43]. Reproduced with permission of Elsevier.

fistulae have a single external opening, have no associated abscess, and begin low in the anorectum. In contrast, a complex fistula is associated with an abscess, begins high in the rectal canal, has multiple openings, or may connect to an adjacent structure such as the vagina [33].

There are several modalities available for the diagnosis of perianal fistulae and associated complications. Traditionally, the first step has involved an exam under anesthesia (EUA). This allows for identification of all fistula tracts, drainage of abscesses, fistulectomy, or placing of a seton as indicated [34]. A CT scan is sometimes helpful to diagnose pelvic abscesses and penetrating complications related to fistulae, but usually has poor accuracy for perianal disease owing to inadequate resolution. Endoscopic ultrasound (EUS) and MRI may have superior utility for perianal CD. On EUS, fistulae are visualized as hypoechoic structures with hyperechogenicity where there is gas within the fistula. An abscess is visualized as a hypoechoic

mass in the perianal region. EUS is superior to a CT scan for the diagnosis of perianal CD but relies on operator experience. Dedicated pelvic MRI is also highly accurate in defining perianal fistulizing disease [35] (Figure 13.5). Institutional preference and experience often dictate the choice of modality for initial evaluation of perianal disease.

Treatment of fistulae depends on three factors: type of fistula, presence of associated abscess, and concomitant luminal inflammatory disease. Antibiotics are very effective in the treatment of perianal CD, particularly in the setting of perianal sepsis and abscess. The most common initial antibiotic choices are ciprofloxacin and metronidazole. Superficial abscesses can be treated by soaking the area in warm water or Sitz baths, which promote drainage. Suspicion for deeper or refractory abscesses should trigger imaging. Deep pelvic or perirectal abscesses may require interventional or operative drainage in conjunction with

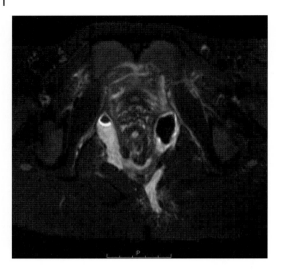

**Figure 13.5** An axial T2 fat-suppressed image showing a trans-sphincteric fistula with a horseshoe abscess and also an additional abscess extending posteriorly into the left ischioanal fossa.

antibiotic therapy. Following treatment of the acute perianal sepsis, patients should begin thiopurine or biologic therapy. Evidence supporting a role for thiopurine therapy is mostly from *post hoc* analysis of trials of azathioprine or 6-mercaptopurine in luminal CD. In a small prospective trial of 52 patients treated with antibiotics, a subset of whom were initiated on azathioprine, response was noted in 48% of those who received azathioprine compared with 15% in those without immunosuppression [36]. In a longer term study, the probability of remaining free of perianal complication with azathioprine at 3 years was 0.47 [37].

In a trial by Present *et al.*, the loading dosing of infliximab 5 mg kg$^{-1}$ at weeks 0, 2, and 6 was associated with a 50% reduction in the number of draining fistulae in 68% of patients [38]. Among those who responded, continued maintenance therapy was associated with a longer time to loss of response (40 weeks) compared with placebo (14 weeks), and a greater proportion of patients achieved complete absence of draining fistulae (36% vs. 19%). Subgroup analysis of the CHARM trial revealed adalimumab to also be efficacious in the treatment of perianal fistulae. Fistula healing was

seen in 33% of patients treated with adalimumab compared with 13% of patients treated with placebo. Further follow-up revealed that fistula closure was durable in 60% at 2 years. There are fewer data regarding the effect of certolizumab pegol on perianal fistulae, although an analysis of the PRECISE 2 data suggest similar efficacy. Combined medical and surgical therapy is associated with greater rates of response and lower rates of recurrence than with medical therapy alone.. In a retrospective study of 32 patients with perianal CD, patients who had an EUA prior to infliximab had a better initial response (100%) and lower recurrence rate (44%) than those who were treated with infliximab alone (initial response 83%, recurrence rate 79%) [39]. Serial imaging with MRI or EUS to assess the response of fistulae may be useful to guide escalation of therapy [40, 41].

Between 25 and 71% of patients with perianal CD require surgery. The range of surgical intervention includes EUA, placement of a seton, abscess drainage, fistulotomy, fistula plugs, advancement flags, temporary or permanent fecal diversion, and proctectomy. The goals of surgical therapy are to eliminate active disease, drain loculated perianal sepsis, and prevent recurrence while maintaining sphincter function. The most commonly performed treatment is EUA with seton placement, where a suture or loop is threaded through the fistula tract and tied outside the anal canal, allowing for continued drainage as the inflammation associated with the tract resolves. Asymptomatic enteroenteric fistulae do not need a change in the medical management other than adequate titration of therapy to control luminal disease. Symptomatic fistulae, enterocutaneous fistulae, or fistulae to other organ systems may require complete bowel rest and total parenteral nutrition. Postoperative fistulae represent a challenging dilemma as in some patients it is difficult to establish if the fistulae are consequent to a post-surgical leak or recurrent CD. If the fistulae develop soon after surgery and appear to arise at the site of the anastomosis, then the cause is likely the former. Poor nutritional status, corticosteroid use, and extensive luminal inflammation with connected bowel loops due to active inflammation increase the risk of postoperative leaks. Often, such leaks need surgical management, although anecdotal reports have attempted endoscopic closure of leaks when visible. Fistulae occurring at the anastomotic site several months after surgery should prompt evaluation for recurrent CD. The response rate for rectovaginal and internal fistulae is lower, and such fistulae usually require surgical treatment, often involving resection of the involved segment of bowel and repair of adjacent organs (e.g., bladder), and temporary or permanent fecal diversion. Even though temporary diversion may be helpful in "cooling down" the disease, recurrence of the fistula on reversal of the stoma is common.

### Small-bowel Cancer

Small-bowel CD is associated with an increased risk of small-bowel adenocarcinoma, with an incidence of 0.46 per 1000 patient-years after 8 years of disease, representing a 30–40-fold increase in incidence compared with the general population. The overall magnitude of small-bowel adenocarcinoma risk is about 30% of the colorectal cancer risk in colonic CD [42]. Routine surveillance for small-bowel cancer with cross-sectional imaging or capsule endoscopy is not warranted.

## Case Studies and Multiple Choice Questions

1   Maria is a 32-year-old woman who reports symptoms of constipation and rectal bleeding. A colonoscopy revealed erythema and granularity in the rectum but it was otherwise normal, including a normal terminal ileum. Biopsies reveal chronic active inflammation in the rectum and no evidence of colitis more proximally. Which of the following statements is true about Maria's disease?

   A  Maria's two children should undergo colonoscopy at age 30 years to screen for ulcerative colitis.

   B  Maria should begin surveillance for colorectal cancer beginning at 15 years after diagnosis and annually thereafter.

   C  Maria should begin surveillance colonoscopies at age 50 years and undergo them every 5–10 years.

   D  Annual fecal occult blood testing should be adopted to screen for colorectal cancer.

2   Which of the following statements is true about *Clostridium difficile* infection in patients with inflammatory bowel diseases?

   A  Patients with IBD are at an increased risk for both infection and adverse outcomes due to *C. difficile* infection.

   B  Pseudomembranes are seen in nearly all patients with IBD who develop *C. difficile* infection.

   C  Most patients with IBD who develop *C. difficile* do so in the setting of recent antibiotic utilization.

   D  Patients with a J-pouch are not at risk for *C. difficile* infection because of the lack of a colon.

3   Which of the following agents have no role in the management of perianal Crohn's disease?

   A  Systemic corticosteroids.

   B  Antibiotics.

   C  Azathioprine.

   D  Anti-TNF biologics.

4   Marjorie is a 48-year-old woman with longstanding Crohn's disease involving the colon. She is currently on treatment with azathioprine 150 mg per day. Of late, over the past 3 months, she has noticed feculent drainage through her vagina. Which of the following statements is true?

   A  The best modality to establish a diagnosis is a colonoscopy.

   B  A CT of the abdomen and pelvis has high sensitivity and specificity in establishing a diagnosis.

   C  MRI of the pelvis should be performed to define the presence of a fistula.

   D  Urinalysis is likely to reveal polymicrobial bacteruria.

5  You obtain a pelvic MRI scan that reveals the presence of a rectovaginal fistula. Which of the following statements is correct?

A  Response to infliximab is likely to be similar to that for perianal fistulae.

B  Marjorie may need colonic diversion to achieve control.

C  Endoscopic therapy is often successful in closing rectovaginal fistulae and should be first line.

D  Mesalamine agents should be first-line treatment for rectovaginal fistula.

# References

1 Ananthakrishnan, A.N., Issa, M., and Binion, D.G. (2010) *Clostridium difficile* and inflammatory bowel disease. *Medical Clinics of North America*, **94**(1), 135–153.

2 Ananthakrishnan, A.N., McGinley, E.L., and Binion, D.G. (2008) Excess hospitalisation burden associated with *Clostridium difficile* in patients with inflammatory bowel disease. *Gut*, **57**(2), 205–210.

3 Ananthakrishnan, A.N., Issa, M., and Binion, D.G. (2009) *Clostridium difficile* and inflammatory bowel disease. *Gastroenterology Clinics of North America*, **38**(4), 711–728.

4 Kandiel, A. and Lashner, B. (2006) Cytomegalovirus colitis complicating inflammatory bowel disease. *American Journal of Gastroenterology*, **101**(12), 2857–2865.

5 Lawlor, G. and Moss, A.C. (2010) Cytomegalovirus in inflammatory bowel disease: pathogen or innocent bystander? *Inflammatory Bowel Diseases*, **16**(9), 1620–1627.

6 Eaden, J.A., Abrams, K.R., and Mayberry, J.F. (2001) The risk of colorectal cancer in ulcerative colitis: a meta-analysis. *Gut*, **48**(4), 526–535.

7 Beaugerie, L., Svrcek, M., Seksik, P., *et al.* (2013) Risk of colorectal high-grade dysplasia and cancer in a prospective observational cohort of patients with inflammatory bowel disease. *Gastroenterology*, **145**(1), 166–175.e8.

8 Jess, T., Simonsen, J., Jorgensen, K.T., *et al.* (2012) Decreasing risk of colorectal cancer in patients with inflammatory bowel disease over 30 years. *Gastroenterology*, **143**(2), 375–381.e1; quiz, e13–14.

9 Jess, T., Rungoe, C., and Peyrin-Biroulet, L. (2012) Risk of colorectal cancer in patients with ulcerative colitis: a meta-analysis of population-based cohort studies. *Clinical Gastroenterology and Hepatology*, **10**(6), 639–645.

10 Friedman, S., Rubin, P.H., Bodian, C., *et al.* (2001) Screening and surveillance colonoscopy in chronic Crohn's colitis. *Gastroenterology*, **120**(4), 820–826.

11 Rubin, D.T., Huo, D., Kinnucan, J.A., *et al.* (2013) Inflammation is an independent risk factor for colonic neoplasia in patients with ulcerative colitis: a case–control study. *Clinical Gastroenterology and Hepatology*, **11**(12), 1601–1608.e1–4.

12 Gupta, R.B., Harpaz, N., Itzkowitz, S., *et al.* (2007) Histologic inflammation is a risk factor for progression to colorectal neoplasia in ulcerative colitis: a cohort study. *Gastroenterology*, **133**(4), 1099–1105; quiz, 340–341.

13 Farraye, F.A., Odze, R.D., Eaden, J., and Itzkowitz, S.H. (2010) AGA technical review on the diagnosis and management of colorectal neoplasia in inflammatory bowel disease. *Gastroenterology*, **138**(2), 746–774.e4; quiz e12–13.

14 Rutter, M.D., Saunders, B.P., Schofield, G., *et al.* (2004) Pancolonic indigo carmine

dye spraying for the detection of dysplasia in ulcerative colitis. *Gut*, **53**(2), 256–260.

15 Ullman, T.A., Loftus, E.V., Jr., Kakar, S., *et al.* (2002) The fate of low grade dysplasia in ulcerative colitis. *American Journal of Gastroenterology*, **97**(4), 922–927.

16 Zisman, T.L., Bronner, M.P., Rulyak, S., *et al.* (2012) Prospective study of the progression of low-grade dysplasia in ulcerative colitis using current cancer surveillance guidelines. *Inflammatory Bowel Diseases*, **18**(12), 2240–2246.

17 Pekow, J.R., Hetzel, J.T., Rothe, J.A., *et al.* (2010) Outcome after surveillance of low-grade and indefinite dysplasia in patients with ulcerative colitis. *Inflammatory Bowel Diseases*, **16**(8), 1352–1356.

18 Ullman, T., Croog, V., Harpaz, N., *et al.* (2003) Progression of flat low-grade dysplasia to advanced neoplasia in patients with ulcerative colitis. *Gastroenterology*, **125**(5), 1311–1319.

19 Rubin, D.T., LoSavio, A., Yadron, N., *et al.* (2006) Aminosalicylate therapy in the prevention of dysplasia and colorectal cancer in ulcerative colitis. *Clinical Gastroenterology and Hepatology*, **4**(11), 1346–1350.

20 van Staa, T.P., Card, T., Logan, R.F., and Leufkens, H.G. (2005) 5-Aminosalicylate use and colorectal cancer risk in inflammatory bowel disease: a large epidemiological study. *Gut*, **54**(11), 1573–1578.

21 Velayos, F.S., Terdiman, J.P., and Walsh, J.M. (2005) Effect of 5-aminosalicylate use on colorectal cancer and dysplasia risk: a systematic review and metaanalysis of observational studies. *American Journal of Gastroenterology*, **100**(6), 1345–1353.

22 Bernstein, C.N., Nugent, Z., and Blanchard, J.F. (2011) 5-Aminosalicylate is not chemoprophylactic for colorectal cancer in IBD: a population based study. *American Journal of Gastroenterology*, **106**(4), 731–736.

23 Nguyen, G.C., Gulamhusein, A., and Bernstein, C.N. (2012) 5-Aminosalicylic acid is not protective against colorectal cancer in inflammatory bowel disease: a meta-analysis of non-referral populations. *American Journal of Gastroenterology*, **107**(9), 1298–1304; quiz, 1297, 1305.

24 Pardi, D.S., Loftus, E.V., Jr., Kremers, W.K., *et al.* (2003) Ursodeoxycholic acid as a chemopreventive agent in patients with ulcerative colitis and primary sclerosing cholangitis. *Gastroenterology*, **124**(4), 889–893.

25 Singh, S., Khanna, S., Pardi, D.S., *et al.* (2013) Effect of ursodeoxycholic acid use on the risk of colorectal neoplasia in patients with primary sclerosing cholangitis and inflammatory bowel disease: a systematic review and meta-analysis. *Inflammatory Bowel Diseases*, **19**(8), 1631–1638.

26 Eaton, J.E., Silveira, M.G., Pardi, D.S., *et al.* (2011) High-dose ursodeoxycholic acid is associated with the development of colorectal neoplasia in patients with ulcerative colitis and primary sclerosing cholangitis. *American Journal of Gastroenterology*, **106**(9), 1638–1645.

27 Wibmer, A.G., Kroesen, A.J., Grone, J., *et al.* (2010) Comparison of strictureplasty and endoscopic balloon dilatation for stricturing Crohn's disease – review of the literature. *International Journal of Colorectal Disease*, **25**(10), 1149–1157.

28 Di Nardo, G., Oliva, S., Passariello, M., *et al.* (2010) Intralesional steroid injection after endoscopic balloon dilation in pediatric Crohn's disease with stricture: a prospective, randomized, double-blind, controlled trial. *Gastrointestinal Endoscopy*, **72**(6), 1201–1208.

29 Swaminath, A. and Lichtiger, S. (2008) Dilation of colonic strictures by intralesional injection of infliximab in patients with Crohn's colitis. *Inflammatory Bowel Diseases*, **14**(2), 213–216.

30 Nguyen, D.L., Sandborn, W.J., Loftus, E.V., Jr., *et al.* (2012) Similar outcomes of surgical and medical treatment of intra-abdominal abscesses in patients with Crohn's disease. *Clinical Gastroenterology and Hepatology*, **10**(4), 400–404.

31 Cullen, G., Vaughn, B., Ahmed, A., *et al.* (2012) Abdominal phlegmons in Crohn's disease: outcomes following antitumor necrosis factor therapy. *Inflammatory Bowel Diseases*, **18**(4), 691–696.

32 Schwartz, D.A., Loftus, E.V., Jr., Tremaine, W.J., *et al.* (2002) The natural history of fistulizing Crohn's disease in Olmsted County, Minnesota. *Gastroenterology*, **122**(4), 875–880.

33 Sandborn, W.J., Fazio, V.W., Feagan, B.G., and Hanauer, S.B. (2003) AGA technical review on perianal Crohn's disease. *Gastroenterology*, **125**(5), 1508–1530.

34 Wise, P.E. and Schwartz, D.A. (2012) The evaluation and treatment of Crohn perianal fistulae: EUA, EUS, MRI, and other imaging modalities. *Gastroenterology Clinics of North America*, **41**(2), 379–391.

35 Schwartz, D.A., Wiersema, M.J., Dudiak, K.M., *et al.* (2001) A comparison of endoscopic ultrasound, magnetic resonance imaging, and exam under anesthesia for evaluation of Crohn's perianal fistulas. *Gastroenterology*, **121**(5), 1064–1072.

36 Dejaco, C., Harrer, M., Waldhoer, T., *et al.* (2003) Antibiotics and azathioprine for the treatment of perianal fistulas in Crohn's disease. *Alimentary Pharmacology & Therapeutics*, **18**(11–12), 1113–1120.

37 Lecomte, T., Contou, J.F., Beaugerie, L., *et al.* (2003) Predictive factors of response of perianal Crohn's disease to azathioprine or 6-mercaptopurine. *Diseases of the Colon and Rectum*, **46**(11), 1469–1475.

38 Present, D.H., Rutgeerts, P., Targan, S., *et al.* (1999) Infliximab for the treatment of fistulas in patients with Crohn's disease. *New England Journal of Medicine*, **340**(18), 1398–1405.

39 Regueiro, M. and Mardini, H. (2003) Treatment of perianal fistulizing Crohn's disease with infliximab alone or as an adjunct to exam under anesthesia with seton placement. *Inflammatory Bowel Diseases*, **9**(2), 98–103.

40 Spradlin, N.M., Wise, P.E., Herline, A.J., *et al.* (2008) A randomized prospective trial of endoscopic ultrasound to guide combination medical and surgical treatment for Crohn's perianal fistulas. *American Journal of Gastroenterology*, **103**(10), 2527–2535.

41 Ng, S.C., Plamondon, S., Gupta, A., *et al.* (2009) Prospective evaluation of anti-tumor necrosis factor therapy guided by magnetic resonance imaging for Crohn's perineal fistulas. *American Journal of Gastroenterology*, **104**(12), 2973–2986.

42 Elriz, K., Carrat, F., Carbonnel, F, *et al.* (2013) Incidence, presentation, and prognosis of small bowel adenocarcinoma in patients with small bowel Crohn's disease: a prospective observational study. *Inflammatory Bowel Diseases*, **19**(9), 1823–1826.

43 Schwartz, D.A. and Maltz, B.E. (2009) Treatment of fistulizing inflammatory bowel disease. *Gastroenterology Clinics of North America*, **38**(4), 595–610.

## Answers to Questions

1   Answer: **C**. Patients with ulcerative proctitis without any proximal extension are not at elevated risk for colorectal cancer and can be entered in a screening program suitable for average-risk individuals without ulcerative colitis. Fecal occult blood testing does not have demonstrated efficacy as a modality for colorectal cancer screening in patients with IBD. There is also no evidence-based justification to screen asymptomatic family members for underlying IBD.

2   Answer: **A**. Patients with IBD are an increased risk for *C. difficile* infection, which in turn is associated with a fourfold increase in mortality. In contrast to individuals without IBD, pseudomembranes are infrequently seen in those with IBD, particularly in the setting of immunosuppression. In addition, over half of the patients with IBD who develop *C. difficile* infection have no other risk factors such as antibiotic use or recent hospitalization. *C. difficile* infections have also been reported in patients with a J-pouch and with an ileostomy. Hence suspicion for this infection must be entertained even in those without an intact colon.

3   Answer: **A**. Systemic corticosteroids are not effective in the management of perianal Crohn's disease and should not be used to treat this complication. Antibiotics are the first-line treatment for perianal fistulae and abscesses in Crohn's disease. There is strong evidence supporting a benefit to using azathioprine or anti-TNF biologics in achieving fistula healing in Crohn's disease, although the effect of the former is more modest than the latter.

4   Answer: **C**. A pelvic MRI study or EUS, with the choice guided by institutional experience and expertise, is the best modality to visualize perianal Crohn's disease. Both a CT scan and a colonoscopy have lower sensitivity in documenting the presence of rectovaginal fistulae. Rectovaginal fistulae are not commonly accompanied by enterovesical fistulae and Marjorie's urinalysis is likely to be normal.

5   Answer: **B**. Unfortunately, internal fistulae often respond poorly to medical therapy and have lower rates of response than perianal or luminal Crohn's disease. Temporary or permanent surgical diversion is often required to achieve control of perianal sepsis. Endoscopic therapy has not been demonstrated to be consistently effective in treating internal rectovaginal fistulae.

Section IV

Special Considerations

# 14

# Nutrition in Inflammatory Bowel Diseases

---

## Clinical Take Home Messages

- Malnutrition and deficiency of micronutrients are common in patients with inflammatory bowel disease (IBD).
- Specific micronutrient deficiencies may result from disease or surgeries in patients with Crohn's Disease (CD). Patients with ileal CD or who have undergone distal ileal resection have more frequent deficiency of vitamin $B_{12}$ and malabsorption of fat-soluble vitamins due to bile salt depletion.

- Low vitamin D may be linked to more severe disease and increase risk for hospitalizations and surgeries.
- Dietary manipulation to achieve disease remission and relief of symptoms is a frequently voiced patient interest. However, there have been few rigorous studies examining dietary interventions in the management of IBD. Elemental diets are effective in inducing remission in pediatric CD but may be inferior to corticosteroids.

---

## Malnutrition and Micronutrient Deficiencies

Malnutrition and deficiency of micronutrients are common in patients with inflammatory bowel disease (IBD), with several contributory reasons. First, gastrointestinal symptoms may interfere with appetite and reduce intake of food. Increased caloric requirements due to catabolism associated with active inflammation may not be met by a corresponding increase in oral intake. Anorexia also occurs as a result of inflammation, side effects of medication, or depression, which is more common in patients with IBD. Second, intolerance to food because of underlying inflammation or a history of surgical resection may result in a restricted diet, leading to

deficiency of nutrients. Third, luminal inflammation interferes with absorption of nutrients in the proximal and distal small intestine, leading to malnutrition. Fistulae contribute to malabsorption by bypassing segments of the gastrointestinal tract. Repeated extensive bowel resections reduce the intestinal absorptive surface area.

Specific micronutrient deficiencies result from both disease and surgeries in patients with Crohn's disease (CD) (Table 14.1). Vitamin $B_{12}$ is mainly absorbed in the distal ileum; patients with ileal CD or who have undergone distal ileal resection have more frequent deficiency of vitamin $B_12$. Interruption of the enterohepatic circulation as a result of ileal resection leads to bile salt malabsorption and a resultant deficiency in

---

*Inflammatory Bowel Diseases: A Clinician's Guide*, First Edition. Ashwin N. Ananthakrishnan, Ramnik J. Xavier, and Daniel K. Podolsky.

**Table 14.1** Common micronutrient deficiency in inflammatory bowel diseases: causes and treatment.

| Micronutrient | Cause(s) of deficiency | Recommended daily allowance | Treatment of deficiency |
|---|---|---|---|
| Folate | Inadequate diet, malabsorption, medications (methotrexate, sulfasalazine) | 400 µg | 1 mg per day |
| Vitamin $B_{12}$ | Ileal resection, active ileitis | 2.4 µg | 1000 µg IM vitamin $B_{12}$ monthly. Oral or intranasal replacements are also options in selected patients |
| Vitamin A | Inadequate dietary intake, fat malabsorption, bile salt deficiency | 700 µg (women); 900 µg (men) | 10 000 IU per day orally or IM × 10 days |
| Vitamin D | Inadequate dietary intake, reduced sunlight exposure | 200–400 IU | 50 000 IU once per week × 12 weeks; 1000–2000 IU daily |
| Calcium | Inadequate dietary intake, vitamin D deficiency, hypomagnesemia | 1000 mg | 1000–1500 mg per day |
| Magnesium | Inadequate dietary intake, losses in stool | 420 mg (men); 320 mg (women) | 5–20 mmol per day |
| Iron | Chronic blood loss, impaired iron metabolism, inadequate dietary intake | 8 mg (men, women >50 years); 18 mg (women <50 years) | IV iron dosing based on iron deficit and hemoglobin; oral iron, 325 mg per day |
| Zinc | Diarrheal losses, malabsorption | 8–11 mg | 220 mg per day |
| Selenium | Long-term total parenteral nutrition | 55 µg | 100 µg per day × 2–3 weeks |

*Source:* Adapted from Hwang *et al.* 2012 [14]. Reproduced with permission of Wolters Kluwer Health.

fat-soluble vitamins. Bile acid malabsorption presents as diarrhea in the absence of active inflammation in those with ileal resection. This is treated with bile acid-binding resins such as cholestyramine (powder), colestipol, or colesevelam (tablets). Bile acid-binding resins should be avoided in patients with extensive (>100 cm) resection of the ileum as the reason for diarrhea in such patients is malabsorption of fat, which is worsened by bile acid sequestrants. Intestinal loss of protein in the setting of severe inflammation can also contribute to deficiency of zinc and magnesium. Finally, medications themselves can contribute to nutritional deficiency – most commonly folate deficiency with sulfasalazine and methotrexate.

Iron deficiency is common in patients with IBD and is variably due to a mixture of chronic intestinal blood loss, reduced absorption, and reduced oral intake. Although animal models suggested potential aggravation of intestinal inflammation with oral iron, trials in patients with CD demonstrated good response and tolerance to oral supplementation [1]. If such supplementation is not tolerated, particularly in those with significant symptoms, intravenous iron is appropriate. Vitamin D deficiency is also common in patients with IBD, particularly CD. This does not seem to be a consequence of longstanding disease alone, as studies have shown that it may pre-date diagnosis and is common even in recently diagnosed patients [2, 3]. Furthermore, low vitamin D may be linked to more severe disease and increase risk for hospitalizations and surgeries [4]. Vitamin D supplementation may prevent relapses in CD [5]. Hence it is prudent to assess for vitamin D deficiency in patients with IBD and to supplement to normalize levels if necessary.

## Dietary Therapies for Inflammatory Bowel Diseases

There is substantial heterogeneity in tolerance of various diets. Most patients in endoscopic remission should be able to tolerate a normal range of food. In the setting of active luminal inflammation, stricturing disease, or following small bowel resection surgery, patients should avoid fibrous, high-residue foods such as raw fruits and vegetables, nuts, celery, and popcorn. A diagnosis of IBD does not preclude patients from having other gastrointestinal diseases, including celiac disease and lactose intolerance. Persistent gastrointestinal symptoms, particularly after endoscopic remission has been achieved, should trigger investigation for these other etiologies.

Dietary manipulation to achieve disease remission and relief of symptoms is a frequently voiced patient interest. However, there have been few rigorous studies examining dietary interventions in the management of IBD. Most reports of efficacy have been anecdotal and self-selected. Dietary surveys administered to patients reveal a wide range of diets that are tolerated, are considered protective, or are considered triggers for symptomatic relapse [6]. Hence the most important nutritional advice to patients with IBD is to eat a well-balanced diet as tolerated in order to avoid macro- and micronutrient deficiencies.

The most widely studied dietary intervention in IBD is the elemental diet. Elemental diets rely on the principle of low dietary antigenic stimulation and consist of amino acids, monosaccharides, essential fatty acids, vitamins, and minerals. They can be administered either orally or, more frequently, via nasogastric tube owing to poor palatability. They have been studied in both the induction and maintenance of remission in CD. Gorard *et al.* compared 22 patients with CD requiring hospitalization for disease flare treated with an elemental diet with 20 patients treated with prednisone $0.75 \text{ mg kg}^{-1}$ per day [7]. Reduction in disease activity was similar in both groups, with similar decreases in C-reactive protein. However, the probability of remaining in remission at 6 months was lower with the elemental diet than with steroids. Elemental diets tend to be poorly tolerated in the long term. Polymeric diets are better tolerated than elemental diets and demonstrate an 80% rate of remission in newly diagnosed CD, with maintenance of remission over a 15-month period [8]. Dietary n-3 fatty acids have been hypothesized to have an anti-inflammatory effect by competitively inhibiting the pro-inflammatory action of prostaglandins and leukotrienes. Although small studies supported a potential effect in ulcerative colitis [9, 10], large placebo-controlled trials of fish oil in CD did not demonstrate a similar benefit [11].

Long-term parenteral nutrition therapy is used infrequently in patients with CD but may be required in patients who have had multiple intestinal resections and chronic small-intestine obstruction not amenable to surgical resection. The role of total parenteral nutrition in boosting nutritional status prior to surgery or its utility in preventing need for surgery is controversial. Total parenteral nutrition does not reduce rates of colectomy and has not been consistently associated with improved outcomes following surgical procedures. Patients with short bowel syndrome may benefit from the GLP-2 analog, teduglutide, which reduces diarrhea, fecal energy losses, and need for parenteral support [12].

## Case Studies and Multiple Choice Questions

1  Satish is a 15-year-old boy with a recent diagnosis of ileocolonic Crohn's disease, inflammatory phenotype. He was advised by his gastroenterologist to initiate prednisone and 6-mercaptopurine but was concerned about side effects of the immunosuppressive therapy. He is seeking a second opinion and inquires about the role of dietary manipulation in management of Crohn's disease. Which of the following dietary therapies have been proven to be effective in inducing remission in Crohn's disease?

A  Elemental diet.
B  Specific carbohydrate diet.
C  Gluten-free diet.
D  Low-fiber diet.

2  Which of the following statements is true about the management of anemia in patients with inflammatory bowel disease?

A  Recurrence of anemia is common without maintenance iron in patients who require intravenous iron therapy.

B  Oral iron therapy is well tolerated in Crohn's disease and is the first-line therapy for those with moderate to severe anemia.
C  Anemia in Crohn's disease is almost always due to iron deficiency alone.
D  Anemia is equally common in Crohn's disease and ulcerative colitis.

3  Which of the following statement about vitamin D deficiency in patients with inflammatory bowel disease is *not* true?

A  Vitamin D deficiency is a consequence of longstanding bowel inflammation and is not seen in newly diagnosed inflammatory bowel disease.
B  Vitamin D deficiency may precede a diagnosis of Crohn's disease.
C  Low levels of vitamin D are associated with an increased risk of surgeries and hospitalization.
D  Vitamin D supplementation is associated with reduced risk of relapse in patients with Crohn's disease.

# References

1 Gasche, C., Berstad, A., Befrits, R., *et al.* (2007) Guidelines on the diagnosis and management of iron deficiency and anemia in inflammatory bowel diseases. *Inflammatory Bowel Diseases*, **13**(12), 1545–1553.

2 Leslie, W.D., Miller, N., Rogala, L., and Bernstein, C.N. (2008) Vitamin D status and bone density in recently diagnosed inflammatory bowel disease: the Manitoba IBD Cohort Study. *American Journal of Gastroenterology*, **103**(6), 1451–1459.

3 Ananthakrishnan, A.N., Khalili, H., Higuchi, L.M., *et al.* (2012) Higher predicted vitamin D status is associated with reduced risk of Crohn's disease. *Gastroenterology*, **142**(3), 482–489.

4 Ananthakrishnan, A.N., Cagan, A., Gainer, V.S., *et al.* (2013) Normalization of plasma 25-hydroxy vitamin D is associated with reduced risk of surgery in Crohn's disease. *Inflammatory Bowel Diseases*, **19**(9), 1921–1927.

5 Jorgensen, S.P., Agnholt, J., Glerup, H., *et al.* (2010) Clinical trial: vitamin $D_3$ treatment in Crohn's disease – a randomized double-blind placebo-controlled study. *Alimentary Pharmacology & Therapeutics*, **32**(3), 377–383.

6 Zallot, C., Quilliot, D., Chevaux, J.B., *et al.* (2013) Dietary beliefs and behavior among inflammatory bowel disease patients. *Inflammatory Bowel Diseases*, **19**(1), 66–72.

7 Gorard, D.A., Hunt, J.B., Payne-James, J.J., *et al.* (1993) Initial response and subsequent course of Crohn's disease treated with elemental diet or prednisolone. *Gut*, **34**(9), 1198–1202.

8 Day, A.S., Whitten, K.E., Lemberg, D.A., *et al.* (2006) Exclusive enteral feeding as primary therapy for Crohn's disease in Australian children and adolescents: a feasible and effective approach. *Journal of Gastroenterology and Hepatology*, **21**(10), 1609–1614.

9 Varnalidis, I., Ioannidis, O., Karamanavi, E., *et al.* (2011) Omega 3 fatty acids supplementation has an ameliorative effect in experimental ulcerative colitis despite increased colonic neutrophil infiltration. *Revista Española de Enfermedades Digestivas*, **103**(10), 511–518.

10 Uchiyama, K., Nakamura, M., Odahara, S., *et al.* (2010) N-3 polyunsaturated fatty acid diet therapy for patients with inflammatory bowel disease. *Inflammatory Bowel Diseases*, **16**(10), 1696–1707.

11 Feagan, B.G., Sandborn, W.J., Mittmann, U., *et al.* (2008) Omega-3 free fatty acids for the maintenance of remission in Crohn disease: the EPIC Randomized Controlled Trials. *JAMA*, **299**(14), 1690–1697.

12 Jeppesen, P.B., Pertkiewicz, M., Messing, B., *et al.* (2012) Teduglutide reduces need

for parenteral support among patients with short bowel syndrome with intestinal failure. *Gastroenterology*, **143**(6), 1473–1481.e3.

13 Zachos, M., Tondeur, M., and Griffiths, A.M. (2007) Enteral nutritional therapy for induction of remission in Crohn's disease.

*Cochrane Database of Systematic Reviews*, (1), CD000542.

14 Hwang, C., Ross, V., and Mahadevan, U. (2012) Micronutrient deficiencies in inflammatory bowel disease: from A to zinc. *Inflammatory Bowel Diseases*, **18**(10), 1961–1981.

## Answers to Questions

1  Answer: **A.** Elemental diets rely on the principle of low dietary antigenic stimulation and consist of amino acids, monosaccharides, essential fatty acids, vitamins, and minerals. They can be administered either orally or, more frequently owing to poor palatability, via nasogastric tube. They have demonstrated efficacy in induction of remission in pediatric Crohn's disease in randomized controlled trials [13]. Although anecdotal reports suggest a benefit to the specific carbohydrate diet in some patients, this has not been rigorously studied in clinical trials. Gluten-free diet and low-fiber diets have not been prospectively studied in Crohn's disease.

2  Answer: **A.** Anemia is common in patients with Crohn's disease and is often multifactorial, which may reflect some combination of chronic inflammation, iron deficiency due to chronic blood loss, poor nutritional intake, protein-energy malnutrition, and/or vitamin $B_{12}$ deficiency. Oral therapy tends to be poorly tolerated in patients with Crohn's disease and intravenous iron replacement is often required. Patients requiring intravenous iron often need monthly maintenance infusions as recurrence of iron deficiency is common without such treatments. Anemia is more common in patients with Crohn's disease than ulcerative colitis.

3  Answer: **A.** Vitamin D deficiency is common in patients with IBD, particularly Crohn's disease. This does not seem to be a consequence of longstanding disease alone, as studies have shown that it may pre-date diagnosis and is common even in recently diagnosed patients [2, 3]. Furthermore, low vitamin D may be linked to more severe disease and increased risk for hospitalizations and surgeries [4], and vitamin D supplementation may prevent relapses in Crohn's disease [5].

15

# Pregnancy, Conception, and Childbirth

## Clinical Take Home Messages

- Crohn's disease (CD) and ulcerative colitis (UC) are not associated with significant reduction in fertility rates except after total proctocolectomy with ileal pouch–anal anastomosis (IPAA) in women, which may be associated with a reduced rate of spontaneous pregnancy.
- The rates of disease flare in pregnant women with inflammatory bowel disease (IBD) are mostly similar to those in women without IBD, and are strongly influenced by disease activity at the time of conception. Inactive disease at conception is usually associated with continued remission throughout pregnancy. In women with active disease at conception, one-third each will experience improvement, stabilization, or worsening of symptoms during pregnancy.
- The rate of adverse pregnancy outcomes in patients with IBD is similar to, or only modestly greater than, that for women without IBD.

- Methotrexate is contraindicated during pregnancy and should be used with caution in women of childbearing age. Other medications are safe to use during pregnancy and conception in both women and men with IBD.
- All four of the approved anti-tumor necrosis factor alpha (TNF) agents (infliximab, adalimumab, certolizumab pegol, and golimumab) are US Food and Drug Administration (FDA) category B agents, with no data to suggest an increase in adverse outcomes following exposure during pregnancy.
- Vaginal delivery appears to be a safe mode of childbirth for most women with CD or UC, except women with active perianal disease.

Inflammatory bowel disease (IBD) commonly affects women and men during their reproductive years. Consequently, its diagnosis and treatment have important implications for conception, pregnancy, and childbirth.

## Fertility

Infertility refers to the inability or reduced ability to conceive within 1 year of regular intercourse without use of contraceptive methods. Initial studies suggested high rates of infertility, between 32 and 42%, among women with Crohn's disease (CD), but included among these were women who were voluntarily without children.

*Inflammatory Bowel Diseases: A Clinician's Guide*, First Edition. Ashwin N. Ananthakrishnan, Ramnik J. Xavier, and Daniel K. Podolsky.
© 2017 John Wiley & Sons Ltd. Published 2017 by John Wiley & Sons Ltd.

More recent population-based studies have estimated the rates of infertility among women with CD to be 5–14%, similar to the rates in the general population. A recent meta-analysis similarly concluded that the 17–44% reduction in fertility reported in CD was due primarily to voluntary childlessness and not to physiologic reasons related to the disease [1].

Surgical treatment for CD may reduce fertility rates slightly, but this effect is not as significant as in ulcerative colitis (UC), where surgical treatment with a total proctocolectomy and an ileal pouch–anal anastomosis (IPAA) results in a significant reduction in spontaneous pregnancy rates. In a meta-analysis of eight relevant studies, the infertility rate in medically treated UC was 15%, comparable to that in the general population, and following a colectomy with IPAA the infertility rate increased to 48% [2]. Contributing to this decrease in fertility are adhesions from pelvic dissection during proctectomy and creation of the ileal pouch and also injury to the reproductive organs in the pelvis. A similar reduction in fertility in seen after surgery for familial adenomatous polyposis [3]. Laparoscopic IPAA may reduce fertility to a lesser extent. Temporizing approaches such as a subtotal colectomy, rectal stump creation, and ileostomy until childbearing is complete are usually not preferred by patients owing to a reluctance to have a long-term stoma, the potential for stoma-related complications, and difficulty in creating the pouch several years after the initial surgery.

Fewer studies have examined the effect of IBD diagnosis on male fertility. In a recent meta-analysis, an 18–50% reduction in fertility of men with CD was observed but, similarly to the association in women, this seemed to be due primarily to voluntary childlessness rather than physiological infertility. There was no reduction in fertility of men with UC [1].

## Effect of Pregnancy on Disease

The rates of disease flare in pregnant women with IBD are mostly similar to those in women without IBD (20–35% per year), although a few studies have suggested an increase in relapse in the postpartum period [4]. A key determinant of disease activity during pregnancy is disease activity at the time of conception [5]. Among women who are in remission at the time of conception, nearly 80% remain in remission during pregnancy compared with 20% who experience a disease flare [4, 6, 7]. In contrast, among women with active disease at the time of conception, one-third each can be expected to have an improvement in their disease activity, no change, and worsening of their disease activity over the course of their pregnancy [7]. In a prospective European cohort of 209 pregnant women, there was no difference in disease course between pregnant women with CD, either during pregnancy or postpartum, compared with non-pregnant women. In contrast, women with UC had a twofold increase in risk of relapse during pregnancy and a sixfold increase in risk of relapse during the postpartum period [8]. Relapses were primarily in the first or second trimester of pregnancy.

## Effect of Disease on Pregnancy

The rate of adverse pregnancy outcomes in patients with IBD is similar to or only mildly greater than that for women without IBD. Women with UC have a modestly increased rate of preterm [odds ratio (OR) 1.77, 95% confidence interval (CI) 1.54–2.05] and small for gestational age babies (OR 1.27, 95% CI 1.05–1.54) than women without UC [9]. Women with CD have a similar increase in risk of moderate (OR 1.76, 95% CI 1.51–2.05) or very preterm birth (OR 1.86, 95% CI 1.38–2.52) [10]. Women with IBD have an increase in risk of venous thromboembolism, particularly in the setting of active disease during pregnancy. There is a twofold increase in elective cesarean section and a more modest increase in emergent cesarean sections [10, 11]. Severity of disease, duration of IBD, or ongoing treatment for the underlying IBD does not influence outcomes of pregnancy [12].

## Maternal Medication Use During Pregnancy

There is a growing body of literature examining maternal and fetal outcomes following exposure to medications used for the treatment of IBD. In general, most of the medications [except methotrexate and thalidomide, which are US Food and Drug Administration (FDA) category X medications and are contraindicated during pregnancy] are safe and continue to be well tolerated during conception and pregnancy (Table 15.1).

Most 5-aminosalicylates (5-ASAs) are FDA pregnancy category B medications, except Asacol® and Asacol® HD, which are FDA category C owing to the presence of dibutyl phthalate in the medication coating. Studies in which animals were exposed to significantly greater amounts of phthalate than present in the drug coating suggested potential adverse effects on the male reproductive system of the fetus. None of the clinical studies of women exposed to Asacol or another 5-ASA during pregnancy have demonstrated adverse effects potentially related to phthalates. A meta-analysis by Rahimi *et al.* pooled seven studies including 2000 pregnant women with IBD, 642 of whom were on a 5-ASA formulation, and found no increase in congenital anomalies, stillbirth, spontaneous abortion, or

**Table 15.1** Medication categories and safety during pregnancy and breastfeeding.

| Therapy | FDA category during pregnancy | Use while breastfeeding |
|---|---|---|
| 5-Aminosalicylates | B[a] | Safe |
| Sulfasalazine | B | Safe |
| Predniso(lo)ne | C | Low risk at doses ≤20 mg per day |
| Budesonide | B | Safe |
| Thiopurines | D | Likely safe |
| Methotrexate | X | Contraindicated |
| Cyclosporine | C | Contraindicated |
| Tacrolimus | C | Probably safe |
| Thalidomide | X | Contraindicated |
| Infliximab | B | Probably safe |
| Adalimumab | B | Probably safe |
| Certolizumab pegol | B | Probably safe |
| Natalizumab | C | Unknown safety |
| Ciprofloxacin | C | Unknown safety |
| Metronidazole | B | Unknown safety |

[a]Asacol® is labeled FDA category C owing to the content of dibutyl phthalate.

low birth weight in babies born to women on 5-ASAs [13]. Previous studies suggesting an increase in risk of preterm births [14] were limited by the inability to separate the effect of disease activity from medication effects. Sulfasalazine is associated with folate deficiency; consequently, women attempting pregnancy while on sulfasalazine should receive a supplement of 1–2 mg of folic acid daily.

Data regarding the safety of thiopurines [azathioprine (AZA), 6-mercaptopurine (6-MP)] during pregnancy have also been mostly reassuring. Early studies demonstrated a modest increase in congenital anomalies (particularly congenital heart disease), preterm delivery, low birth weight, and small for gestational age babies in women exposed to thiopurine therapy during pregnancy. However, more recent studies have failed to identify such an effect. In the PIANO registry, a prospective cohort of pregnant women followed in the United States, there was no increase in adverse outcomes among babies born to women on thiopurines. The CESAME cohort in France, including 204 women exposed to thiopurines during pregnancy, also found no apparent increase in adverse outcomes in infants born to women receiving thiopurine therapy [15]. Long-term follow-up of such infants for a median of 4 years did not find any differences in medical or psychological health among the children exposed to thiopurines *in utero* [16].

All four of the approved anti-tumor necrosis factor alpha (TNF) agents (infliximab, adalimumab, certolizumab pegol, and golimumab) are FDA category B agents with no data to suggest an increase in adverse outcomes following exposure during pregnancy. Infliximab is an immunoglobulin G1 (IgG1) antibody that is transported across the placenta most efficiently in the third trimester, with some transfer also occurring earlier in the second trimester. Cord blood studies have shown that maternal use of infliximab results

in a detectable serum level in newborns that drops soon after birth. Adalimumab is also an IgG1 antibody, and although there are fewer data on its pharmacodynamics during pregnancy, it likely has a rate of transfer across the placenta similar to that of infliximab. In contrast, certolizumab pegol is a pegylated Fab fragment that does not have the Fc portion required for transplacental transfer. Consequently, it may be the preferred anti-TNF agent to initiate during pregnancy in anti-TNF-naive patients. A systematic review of 58 unique studies of the use of anti-TNF agents in women during pregnancy did not identify any increase in adverse pregnancy outcomes or congenital malformations among infants born to such women, and no increase in infections in the offspring of mothers who had received these agents during pregnancy [17, 18]. The PIANO registry suggested a modest increase in risk of infections in women on combination therapy, although other studies, including a recent systematic review [18], did not identify such an effect. Consequently, anti-TNF agents can be continued during pregnancy and administered through the mid third trimester without clinical implications for the baby except for avoidance of live attenuated vaccines for 6 months following birth.

Corticosteroids are FDA pregnancy category C agents and safe for use during pregnancy. An early study suggested a threefold increase in the risk of orofacial clefts among children born to women exposed to steroids early during pregnancy [19]. Consequently, steroids should be avoided if possible during the first trimester of pregnancy. However, the rate of other adverse outcomes was low. Budesonide use was demonstrated to be safe in a small case series [20]. There are limited data on natalizumab, vedolizumab, and cyclosporine use during pregnancy, but all appear to be safe.

Thalidomide and methotrexate are FDA category X drugs and should not be used in pregnancy. Women of reproductive age should be counseled on the risk of teratogenicity with methotrexate, and its use should be discontinued at least 6 months prior to conception. Ciprofloxacin can cause arthropathy in the baby and should be avoided during pregnancy. Metronidazole should also be avoided during pregnancy owing to increased rates of cleft lip and cleft palate. Penicillins such as amoxicillin are good options for use during pregnancy.

Vaginal delivery appears to be a safe mode of childbirth for most women with CD or UC. There does not appear to be increased risk of new-onset perianal disease or clinically relevant perianal trauma following vaginal delivery. Cesarean section is preferred in those with active perianal disease. Some physicians favor delivery via cesarean section in those with a J-pouch.

Oral 5-ASAs are approved for use during lactation by the American Academy of Pediatrics. The sulfa moiety in sulfasalazine can theoretically lead to neonatal hyperbilirubinemia, although this has not been clinically demonstrated. Corticosteroids are likely secreted in small amounts in breast milk, but currently no formal recommendations exist regarding their use during breastfeeding. In women on doses higher than 20 mg per day, a 4 h delay between corticosteroid intake and breastfeeding has been advised [21]. Limited studies have also shown very low levels of AZA or 6-MP excretion into breast milk. The clinical significance of such transfer is low and thiopurines may be continued during breastfeeding, although theoretical concerns about risk of pancreatitis in the neonate have been expressed. Infliximab, adalimumab, and certolizumab pegol are excreted in very small, clinically insignificant amounts in breast milk and have not been associated with neonatal immunosup-

pression. However, live vaccines should be avoided for the first 6 months in infants born to women on biologic therapy.

## Paternal Medication Use

In men, sulfasalazine can have a detrimental effect on sperm quality and consequently a switch to an alternative 5-ASA preparation should be considered at least 3 months prior to planned conception. Paternal thiopurine use during or prior to pregnancy has not been shown to have any adverse effects [22]. Paternal methotrexate exposure has not been demonstrated to lead to congenital anomalies [23], yet most providers recommend a 3-month drug hiatus prior to conception.

## Inheritance

One of the primary concerns of parents with IBD is the risk of passing on the disease to their children. Family history is a strong predictor for the development of IBD. However, only 10–20% of patients with IBD have an affected first-degree relative [24]. If one parent is affected with IBD, the risk of the offspring developing the disease ranges from 2- to 13-fold the incidence in the general population. This risk increases to as high as 36% if both parents have IBD. The risk of development of IBD, however, varies by both type of IBD and ethnicity. In a large study of 527 patients with IBD, the lifetime risk of developing IBD was 5.2% in relatives of probands with CD compared with 1.6% in those with UC [25]. Both rates were higher (7.8% and 4.5%, respectively) among Jews [25]. (See Chapters 1 and 2 for more details.)

# Case Studies and Multiple Choice Questions

1  Amanda is a 27-year-old woman with a 6-year history of ulcerative colitis. She is currently receiving infliximab 5 mg kg$^{-1}$ every 8 weeks, having previously failed with mesalamine and azathioprine. She is in clinical remission and she and her husband are contemplating pregnancy. Which of the following statements are true about fertility and IBD?

   A  Amanda is likely to have lower rates of conception because of her history of ulcerative colitis.

   B  Amanda is likely to have lower rates of conception because of her use of infliximab.

   C  Amanda can expect similar rates of conception to a healthy individual.

   D  Owing to high risk of ulcerative colitis in her offspring, Amanda should not contemplate conception.

2  She returns for follow-up 9 months later and reports that she is 2 months' pregnant. During this pregnancy, Amanda is more likely to experience which of the following outcomes?

   A  Gestational diabetes.

   B  Preterm delivery.

   C  Minor congenital anomalies.

   D  Spontaneous abortions.

3  Which is the appropriate medical management for Amanda during her pregnancy?

   A  Stop infliximab immediately and monitor for disease relapse during pregnancy and use corticosteroids as needed.

   B  Stop infliximab and switch to adalimumab.

   C  Continue infliximab throughout pregnancy.

   D  Stop infliximab and switch to azathioprine until delivery.

4  If, after this pregnancy, Amanda were to require surgery for management of IBD, which of the following statements is true for subsequent pregnancies?

   A  Both J-pouch surgery and a subtotal colectomy with an ileostomy are associated with similar reduction in fertility in patients with ulcerative colitis.

   B  J-pouch surgery is associated with greater impairment of fertility than a subtotal colectomy with ileostomy.

   C  J-pouch surgery is associated with lower impairment of fertility than a subtotal colectomy with ileostomy.

# References

1 Tavernier, N., Fumery, M., Peyrin-Biroulet, L., *et al.* (2013) Systematic review: fertility in non-surgically treated inflammatory bowel disease. *Alimentary Pharmacology & Therapeutics*, **38**(8), 847–853.

2 Waljee, A., Waljee, J., Morris, A.M., and Higgins, P.D. (2006) Threefold increased risk of infertility: a meta-analysis of infertility after ileal pouch anal anastomosis in ulcerative colitis. *Gut*, **55**(11), 1575–1580.

3 Rajaratnam, S.G., Eglinton, T.W., Hider, P., and Fearnhead, N.S. (2011) Impact of ileal pouch–anal anastomosis on female fertility: meta-analysis and systematic review. *International Journal of Colorectal Disease*, **26**(11), 1365–1374.

4 Nielsen, O.H., Andreasson, B., Bondesen, S., and Jarnum, S. (1983) Pregnancy in ulcerative colitis. *Scandinavian Journal of Gastroenterology*, **18**(6), 735–742.

5 Abhyankar, A., Ham, M., and Moss, A.C. (2013) Meta-analysis: the impact of disease activity at conception on disease activity during pregnancy in patients with inflammatory bowel disease. *Alimentary Pharmacology & Therapeutics*, **38**(5), 460–466.

6 Khosla, R., Willoughby, C.P., and Jewell, D.P. (1984) Crohn's disease and pregnancy. *Gut*, **25**(1), 52–56.

7 Beaulieu, D.B. and Kane, S. (2011) Inflammatory bowel disease in pregnancy. *World Journal of Gastroenterology*, **17**(22), 2696–2701.

8 Pedersen, N., Bortoli, A., Duricova, D., *et al.* (2013) The course of inflammatory bowel disease during pregnancy and postpartum: a prospective European ECCO-EpiCom Study of 209 pregnant women. *Alimentary Pharmacology & Therapeutics*, **38**(5), 501–512.

9 Stephansson, O., Larsson, H., Pedersen, L., *et al.* (2011) Congenital abnormalities and other birth outcomes in children born to women with ulcerative colitis in Denmark and Sweden. *Inflammatory Bowel Diseases*, **17**(3), 795–801.

10 Ng, S.W. and Mahadevan, U. (2013) Management of inflammatory bowel disease in pregnancy. *Expert Review of Clinical Immunology*, **9**(2), 161–173; quiz, 174.

11 Broms, G., Granath, F., Linder, M., *et al.* (2012) Complications from inflammatory bowel disease during pregnancy and delivery. *Clinical Gastroenterology and Hepatology*, **10**(11), 1246–1252.

12 Mahadevan, U., Sandborn, W.J., Li, D.K., *et al.* (2007) Pregnancy outcomes in women with inflammatory bowel disease: a large community-based study from Northern California. *Gastroenterology*, **133**(4), 1106–1112.

13 Rahimi, R., Nikfar, S., Rezaie, A., and Abdollahi, M. (2008) Pregnancy outcome in women with inflammatory bowel disease following exposure to 5-aminosalicylic acid drugs: a meta-analysis. *Reproductive Toxicology (Elmsford, NY)*, **25**(2), 271–275.

14 Norgard, B., Fonager, K., Pedersen, L., *et al.* (2003) Birth outcome in women exposed to 5-aminosalicylic acid during pregnancy: a Danish cohort study. *Gut*, **52**(2), 243–247.

15 Coelho, J., Beaugerie, L., Colombel, J.F., *et al.* (2011) Pregnancy outcome in patients with inflammatory bowel disease treated with thiopurines: cohort from the CESAME Study. *Gut*, **60**(2), 198–203.

16 de Meij, T.G., Jharap, B., Kneepkens, C.M., *et al.* (2013) Long-term follow-up of children exposed intrauterine to maternal thiopurine therapy during pregnancy in females with inflammatory bowel disease. *Alimentary Pharmacology & Therapeutics*, **38**(1), 38–43.

17 Gisbert, J.P. and Chaparro, M. (2013) Safety of anti-TNF agents during pregnancy and breastfeeding in women with inflammatory bowel disease. *American Journal of Gastroenterology*, **108**(9), 1426–1438.

18 Nielsen, O.H., Loftus, E.V., Jr., and Jess, T. (2013) Safety of TNF-α inhibitors during IBD pregnancy: a systematic review. *BMC Medicine*, **11**, 174.

19 Park-Wyllie, L., Mazzotta, P., Pastuszak, A., *et al.* (2000) Birth defects after maternal exposure to corticosteroids: prospective cohort study and meta-analysis of epidemiological studies. *Teratology*, **62**(6), 385–392.

20 Beaulieu, D.B., Ananthakrishnan, A.N., Issa, M., *et al.* (2009) Budesonide induction and maintenance therapy for Crohn's disease during pregnancy. *Inflammatory Bowel Diseases*, **15**(1), 25–28.

21 van der Woude, C.J., Kolacek, S., Dotan, I., *et al.* (2010) European evidenced-based consensus on reproduction in inflammatory bowel disease. *Journal of Crohn's & Colitis*, **4**(5), 493–510.

22 Hoeltzenbein, M., Weber-Schoendorfer, C., Borisch, C., *et al.* (2012) Pregnancy outcome after paternal exposure to azathioprine/6-mercaptopurine. *Reproductive Toxicology (Elmsford, NY)*, **34**(3), 364–369.

23 Beghin, D., Cournot, M.P., Vauzelle, C., and Elefant, E. (2011) Paternal exposure to methotrexate and pregnancy outcomes. *Journal of Rheumatology*, **38**(4), 628–632.

24 Binder, V. and Orholm, M. (1996) Familial occurrence and inheritance studies in inflammatory bowel disease. *Netherlands Journal of Medicine*, **48**(2), 53–56.

25 Yang, H., McElree, C., Roth, M.P., *et al.* (1993) Familial empirical risks for inflammatory bowel disease: differences between Jews and non-Jews. *Gut*, **34**(4), 517–524.

## Answers to Questions

1 Answer: **C**. A diagnosis of ulcerative colitis and medical therapy for ulcerative colitis are not associated with reduced fertility in patients. Even with her history of ulcerative colitis, her offspring carry only a 5–10% lifetime risk of IBD, and this should not represent a contraindication for conception and pregnancy.

2 Answer: **B**. The rate of adverse pregnancy outcomes in patients with IBD is similar to or only slightly higher than that for women without IBD. Women with ulcerative colitis have a modestly increased rate of preterm (OR 1.77, 95% CI 1.54–2.05) and small for gestational age babies (OR 1.27, 95% CI 1.05–1.54) than women without ulcerative colitis [9].

3 Answer: **C**. Both infliximab and adalimumab are IgG1 antibodies and have similar rates of transplacental transfer, hence there is no clinical benefit to switching between these agents and evidence suggests that such a switch, at least in a non-pregnant setting, may be associated with risk of relapse. As adequate control of disease during pregnancy is associated with better maternal and fetal outcomes, cessation of therapy or switching to a previously ineffective drug may increase her risk of relapse during pregnancy. Continuing infliximab therapy during pregnancy is not associated with increased risk of birth defects, low birth weight, or preterm births, hence it can be continued until the mid third trimester.

4 Answer: **B**. A J-pouch surgery following subtotal colectomy is associated with a greater reduction in fertility than a subtotal colectomy and ileostomy in patients with ulcerative colitis.

# 16

# Inflammatory Bowel Disease During Childhood and Adolescence

---

## Clinical Take Home Messages

- Approximately 15% of patients with ulcerative colitis and 25–33% of patients with Crohn's disease present during childhood or adolescence.
- Extension of disease is more common in pediatric inflammatory bowel disease (IBD), as is upper gastrointestinal tract involvement.
- The medical management of pediatric IBD resembles that of adult-onset IBD. However, it is essential to assess the impact of disease on growth,

development, and educational and social performance.
- Very early-onset IBD represents a distinct phenotype that develops in children within the first few months of life and is characterized by pancolonic inflammation and a high frequency of perianal involvement, and is often refractory to medical therapy. In many patients, this phenotype is due to polymorphisms in interleukin-10 or interleukin-10 receptor and responds to allogenic stem-cell transplantation.

---

## Epidemiology and Clinical Features

There has been an increase in the incidence of pediatric inflammatory bowel disease (IBD) over the past few decades [1]. Approximately 15% of patients with ulcerative colitis (UC) and 25–33% of patients with Crohn's disease (CD) present during childhood or adolescence. Pediatric UC resembles adult-onset disease in its symptoms, with rectal bleeding and diarrhea being the dominant symptoms. CD in children can present with the typical features of abdominal pain and diarrhea. However, it can also present subtly in the form of growth failure, weight loss, and delayed maturation.

Indeed, growth failure occurs in 10–56% of pediatric patients with CD compared with 0–10% of those with UC [2]. Distinct differences exist between the epidemiology of pediatric IBD compared with adult-onset disease. Pediatric UC (but not CD) demonstrates a slight male predominance not seen in adults [3]. Children also demonstrate a slight predilection towards CD, with a CD:UC ratio of 2.8:1 [3]. Pediatric CD tends to be ileocolonic or colon-only disease more frequently than adult disease, which frequently affects only the terminal ileum. The disease location tends to be stable in adult CD; in contrast, in 39% of pediatric patients, the anatomic extent increases within 2 years of diagnosis. A panenteric

*Inflammatory Bowel Diseases: A Clinician's Guide*, First Edition. Ashwin N. Ananthakrishnan, Ramnik J. Xavier, and Daniel K. Podolsky.

phenotype (involving the upper gastrointestinal tract) is seen more commonly in pediatric than in adult CD. Pediatric UC also presents with pancolitis more often (80–90% of children) compared with adult disease, which frequently presents as proctitis or left-sided colitis [3]. Extraintestinal manifestations and impaired bone density are more common in pediatric IBD. In addition, pediatric IBD has a significant psychosocial impact on children. Depression and anxiety are more common in children with IBD [4]. The embarrassing nature of the symptoms may be associated with delayed disclosure to others and consequently delay in diagnosis. Disease activity may interfere with maintenance of normal academic functioning and development of interpersonal relationships. Self-management of treatment regimens represents a significant challenge for children with IBD. A focus on psychosocial issues and maintenance of normal functioning are an important part of the management of IBD in pediatric patients.

## Treatment of Pediatric Inflammatory Bowel Disease

The medical management of pediatric IBD generally resembles that of adult-onset IBD. No randomized controlled trials (RCTs) have examined the role of 5-aminosalicylates (5-ASA) in the treatment of IBD in children. Extrapolating from meta-analyses examining their efficacy in adults, there does not appear to be a significant role for 5-ASA in the management of pediatric CD. In contrast, randomized trials in adults support significant efficacy for the use of 5-ASA in the induction and management of remission in UC. Owing to their effect on epiphyseal plate closure and association with impaired bone mineral density, corticosteroids should be used sparingly in the management of pediatric IBD. RCTs support the efficacy of thiopurines in the maintenance of remission

and a reduction in the need for corticosteroids. In a landmark trial, Markowitz et al. randomized 55 children with newly diagnosed moderate to severe CD to either 6-mercaptopurine (6-MP) (1.5 mg kg$^{-1}$) or placebo in addition to 40 mg per day of prednisone, tapered on a predefined schedule. At the end of the trial, only 9% of patients in the 6-MP group relapsed compared with 47% in the placebo arm [5]. Other studies have also supported early immunomodulator use in pediatric CD with reduction in the corticosteroid exposure and fewer hospitalizations [6]. The REACH study group evaluated the efficacy and safety of infliximab in the management of children with moderate to severe CD. After receiving the initial induction dosing of 5 mg kg$^{-1}$ at 0, 2, and 6 weeks, 112 children were randomized to infliximab 5 mg kg$^{-1}$ every 8 or 12 weeks through week 46. At week 10, 88% of patients responded to infliximab and 59% achieved clinical remission, rates much higher than reported from adult infliximab trials [7]. Longer term follow-up studies demonstrated that up to 67% of patients are able to maintain the treatment 3 years after infusion. Similarly to that observed in adults, early treatment of pediatric CD yields greater response rates than that found in late disease [8]. The IMAgINE 1 study evaluated the safety and efficacy of adalimumab in pediatric CD. A total of 192 patients were randomized to 40 mg (or 20 mg for body weight below 40 kg$^{-1}$) or 20 mg (10 mg for body weight below 40 kg$^{-1}$) of adalimumab every 2 weeks. At 26 weeks, one-third of the patients were in clinical remission, with a safety profile similar to that seen in adults [9]. Neither the infliximab nor the adalimumab trials in children had a placebo arm. Certolizumab pegol, golimumab, natalizumab, and vedolizumab have not been evaluated in pediatric patients. Hyams et al. conducted an RCT examining the efficacy of infliximab in UC [10]. After standard induction dosing, 73% of pediatric patients with UC achieved a response at week 8; the remission rate at 54 weeks was 38% in the every-8-weeks maintenance arm and 18% in the every-12-weeks maintenance arm, suggesting that the maintenance dosing schedule for infliximab in pediatric patients with UC should be similar to that in adults.

Several studies have examined the efficacy of enteral nutrition therapy in the management of pediatric CD. Borrelli *et al.* performed a prospective 10-week open-label trial comparing polymeric formula with oral corticosteroids in 37 children with active CD. At week 10, a larger proportion of children in the polymeric diet group demonstrated mucosal healing compared with those in the corticosteroid arm, despite similar rates of clinical remission [11]. However, a Cochrane review including adult nutritional therapy trials concluded that corticosteroid therapy was more effective than nutritional therapy for inducing remission [12, 13]. An exclusive elemental diet, even for only 6–8 weeks, to induce remission tends to be poorly tolerated by children and often requires nocturnal administration via nasogastric or gastrostomy tubes.

## Very Early-onset Inflammatory Bowel Disease

Very early-onset IBD represents a distinct phenotype in which IBD develops in children within the first few months of life. This phenotype is usually associated with pancolonic inflammation and a high frequency of perianal involvement, often refractory to medical therapy. Glocker *et al.* performed genetic-linkage analysis and candidate gene sequencing in nine patients with early-onset disease and identified three distinct homozygous mutations in genes *IL10RA* and *IL10RB* in the interleukin-10 receptor [14]. One patient underwent an allogenic hematopoietic stem-cell transplant that resulted in clinical remission. Other studies have subsequently

replicated this association in larger series, confirming sustained clinical remission after allogenic stem-cell transplantation [15].

## Transition of Care in Pediatric Crohn's Disease

Transition of care, defined as "the purposeful, planned movement of adolescents and young adults with chronic health conditions from pediatric to adult care," is a critical time in the course of the patient with pediatric IBD. There is significant heterogeneity in the readiness of pediatric patients with IBD to transition care with regard to their developmental maturity, parental and other family support, and understanding of disease. This represents a particularly challenging time, with a higher likelihood of non-adherence to treatment and discontinuity of care. Demands posed by school or new enrollment in a college distant from home may also adversely impact healthcare behavior during this period.

Barriers to a successful transition may lie with the patient, the provider, or the health-system infrastructure (Table 16.1). Patients with IBD diagnosed at a young age and/or those who had less involvement in medication decisions had significantly more negative experience with transition [16]. Relatively few adult providers feel competent in addressing development issues or the specific medical needs of adolescents. System-based barriers can include incomplete transfer of medical history, including medication regimens.

The physical structure of pediatric practices usually differs from that of adult practices, which may be less likely to incorporate multidisciplinary teams or be based at a specialist center. Additionally, specific diagnostic procedure-related risks such as radiation exposure with radiologic investigations, or risks associated with therapy, such as hepatosplenic T-cell lymphoma related to

**Table 16.1** Barriers to successful transition of care of adolescents with inflammatory bowel disease.

| Factors | Contributing barriers |
|---|---|
| Patient-related factors | Anxiety and depression are more common in pediatric IBD |
| | Demands related to school exams, higher education, and employment, often impacting adherence and continuation of care |
| | Inadequate understanding regarding disease in pediatric IBD |
| | Less understanding regarding consequences of non-adherence in pediatric IBD |
| | Passive role in decision-making and parental influence is more common in pediatric IBD |
| Provider related factors | Inadequate training among adult gastroenterologists regarding screening and treatment of growth failure, developmental delay |
| | Failure to recognize differences in disease phenotype (more common occurrence of Crohn's disease, greater frequency of pancolitis) or treatment-related side effects (effect of prednisone on epiphyseal plate closure, hepatosplenic T-cell lymphoma with thiopurine or combination therapy) |
| | Variations in investigation protocols (risks related to radiation from computed tomography or X-ray imaging; use of general anesthesia for endoscopic procedures) |
| System-related factors | Less frequent availability of multidisciplinary support |
| | Shorter appointment duration in adult IBD |

combination immunosuppression or thiopurine therapy, may be more pertinent to adolescents or young adults with IBD. Practices have adopted different models for successful transition. Care during the transition period typically occurs in the adult practice setting but in conjunction with both the primary pediatric gastroenterologist and new adult provider. A multidisciplinary approach by the transition team also facilitates successful transition, in particular inclusion of nutritionist or dieticians and psychologists. The period of transition care may be variable, but is usually over two or more visits.

## Case Studies and Multiple Choice Questions

1  Which of the following statements is *not* true about pediatric-onset inflammatory bowel disease?
   A  Ileal-only Crohn's disease is more common than Crohn's disease in pediatric patients.
   B  Extraintestinal symptoms are more frequent in pediatric IBD than adult IBD.
   C  Pancolitis is more common in pediatric than adult-onset ulcerative colitis.
   D  Pan-gastrointestinal tract involvement is more common in pediatric Crohn's disease than adult-onset disease.

2  Which of the following mutations have been associated with very early onset IBD?

A  *NOD2.*
B  *ATG16L1.*
C  *IL23R.*
D  *IL10R.*

3  Which of the following side effects are observed more commonly in pediatric and young adult patients compared than in older adult patients on combination immunosuppression therapy for Crohn's disease?
   A  Hepatosplenic T-cell lymphoma.
   B  Non-melanoma skin cancer.
   C  Anti-TNF-related psoriasis.
   D  *Pneumocystis jiroveci* pneumonia.

# References

1 Benchimol, E.I., Fortinsky, K.J., Gozdyra, P., *et al.* (2011) Epidemiology of pediatric inflammatory bowel disease: a systematic review of international trends. *Inflammatory Bowel Diseases*, **17**(1), 423–439.

2 Abraham, B.P., Mehta, S., and El-Serag, H.B. (2012) Natural history of pediatric-onset inflammatory bowel disease: a systematic review. *Journal of Clinical Gastroenterology*, **46**(7), 581–589.

3 Van Limbergen, J., Russell, R.K., Drummond, H.E., *et al.* (2008) Definition of phenotypic characteristics of childhood-onset inflammatory bowel disease. *Gastroenterology*, **135**(4), 1114–1122.

4 Loftus, E.V., Jr., Guerin, A., Yu, A.P., *et al.* (2011) Increased risks of developing anxiety and depression in young patients with Crohn's disease. *American Journal of Gastroenterology*, **106**(9), 1670–1677.

5 Markowitz, J., Grancher, K., Kohn, N., *et al.* (2000) A multicenter trial of 6-mercaptopurine and prednisone in children with newly diagnosed Crohn's disease. *Gastroenterology*, **119**(4), 895–902.

6 Punati, J., Markowitz, J., Lerer, T., *et al.* (2008) Effect of early immunomodulator use in moderate to severe pediatric Crohn disease. *Inflammatory Bowel Diseases*, **14**(7), 949–954.

7 Hyams, J., Crandall, W., Kugathasan, S., *et al.* (2007) Induction and maintenance infliximab therapy for the treatment of moderate-to-severe Crohn's disease in children. *Gastroenterology*, **132**(3), 863–873; quiz, 1165–1166.

8 Kugathasan, S., Werlin, S.L., Martinez, A., *et al.* (2000) Prolonged duration of response to infliximab in early but not late pediatric Crohn's disease. *American Journal of Gastroenterology*, **95**(11), 3189–3194.

9 Hyams, J.S., Griffiths, A., Markowitz, J., *et al.* (2012) Safety and efficacy of adalimumab for moderate to severe Crohn's disease in children. *Gastroenterology*, **143**(2), 365–374.e2.

10 Hyams, J., Damaraju, L., Blank, M., *et al.* (2012) Induction and maintenance therapy with infliximab for children with moderate to severe ulcerative colitis. *Clinical Gastroenterology and Hepatology*, **10**(4), 391–399.e1.

11 Borrelli, O., Cordischi, L., Cirulli, M., *et al.* (2006) Polymeric diet alone versus corticosteroids in the treatment of active pediatric Crohn's disease: a randomized controlled open-label trial. *Clinical Gastroenterology and Hepatology*, **4**(6), 744–753.

12 Zachos, M., Tondeur, M., and Griffiths, A.M. (2007) Enteral nutritional therapy for induction of remission in Crohn's disease. *Cochrane Database of Systematic Reviews*, (1), CD000542.

13 Akobeng, A.K. and Thomas, A.G. (2007) Enteral nutrition for maintenance of remission in Crohn's disease. *Cochrane Database of Systematic Reviews*, (3), CD005984.

14 Glocker, E.O., Kotlarz, D., Boztug, K., *et al.* (2009) Inflammatory bowel disease and

mutations affecting the interleukin-10 receptor. *New England Journal of Medicine*, **361**(21), 2033–2045.

15  Kotlarz, D., Beier, R., Murugan, D., *et al.* (2012) Loss of interleukin-10 signaling and infantile inflammatory bowel disease: implications for diagnosis and therapy. *Gastroenterology*, **143**(2), 347–355.

16  Plevinsky, J.M., Gumidyala, A.P., and Fishman, L.N. (2015) Transition experience of young adults with inflammatory bowel diseases (IBD): a mixed methods study. *Child: Care, Health and Development*, **41**(5), 755–761.

17  Kotlyar, D.S., Osterman, M.T., Diamond, R.H., *et al.* (2011) A systematic review of factors that contribute to hepatosplenic T-cell lymphoma in patients with inflammatory bowel disease. *Clinical Gastroenterology and Hepatology*, **9**(1), 36–41.e1.

## Answers to Questions

1 Answer: **A**. Pediatric CD tends to be ileocolonic or colon-only disease more frequently than adult-onset disease, which frequently affects only the terminal ileum. Pediatric UC also presents more often with pancolitis (80–90% of children) compared with adults in whom proctitis or left-sided colitis is common [3]. Extra-intestinal manifestations and impaired bone density are more common in pediatric IBD.

2 Answer: **D**. Mutations in the interleukin-10 receptor are an important cause of very early-onset IBD (VEOIBD), defined as children who develop the disease before the age of 6–10 years.

This is characterized by frequent colonic involvement in over 80% of individuals, refractoriness to standard therapy, and responsiveness to bone marrow transplantation [14].

3 Answer: **A**. Hepatosplenic T-cell lymphoma is a rare, progressively fatal malignancy observed in individuals using thiopurine monotherapy or in combination with biologics in CD. Although the overall risk of the complication is low (estimated to be 1:22 000), nearly all the cases reported thus far have been in males younger than 35 years of age. The absolute risk in this subgroup is estimated to be 1:3534 with combination therapy [17].

# Index

Page numbers in *italics* refer to illustrations; those in **bold** refer to tables

*Inflammatory Bowel Diseases: A Clinician's Guide*, First Edition. Ashwin N. Ananthakrishnan,
Ramnik J. Xavier, and Daniel K. Podolsky.
© 2017 John Wiley & Sons Ltd. Published 2017 by John Wiley & Sons Ltd.